The Best Body 30 Days Challenges

30 Habit-Forming Programs to Live a Better Life

SUSAN JOHNSON

Table Of Contents

Introduction

What is "Life"? Definitions from dictionaries: The course of existence or sum of experiences and actions that constitute a person's existence. What do YOU think of "life"? How do you live it?

Living a good life comes from happiness and contentment, as the two often go hand in hand. However, we are sometimes looking for happiness from the wrong things and in the wrong places that we end up being frustrated and disappointed.

We may differ in what is a life that is good but there are some important things, big and small, that contributes a lot in what we call living a good life. Here are some tips and ideas that you might find useful in finding ways to have that life that is good we all want to have.

Everybody wants to live a better life, but nobody wants to step up and make it happen for themselves. People make up thousands of excuses as to why they aren't living "the good life". Saying mean things like "I can't have a better life because I wasn't born into a rich family" or "I'm not good looking enough" or "Nothing ever goes my way". Unfortunately not everyone is just born into wealth and luck, but you can have both. Focus on what you want to happen and not what you don't want to happen because that's how to live a better life.

Everyone wants to know how to live a better life. It's a question that cuts across all social classes - from minimum wage employees to famous celebrities. They may not ask it all in the same way, but the underlying question is clear.

How does one live a better life? There's no one answer for that. After all, there are so many factors to consider. First off, you have to define the meaning of a better life. Then, you have to determine the kind of person you are and the realities with which you are surrounded.

In this wonderful guide, we are going to focus on the major things and factors that could make one live a better life.

Chapter 1: Living a Better Life

What Does Good life Mean to You?

The term, "The Good Life" is a very broad concept with a lot of meanings from different people. It may mean a lot of different things to a lot of different people. To me, it simply means a life of blessing and satisfaction. It doesn't mean that you are an important person or that you have a bunch of money. You may be penniless and confined to a wheelchair and living a good life because you are not confined in your mind. You live a good life when you are free.

When I was a child, I would hear the adults refer to "the good life." I didn't think much about it because to me life was already good. I had parents who loved me, friends, school and hours and hours of play. Looking back, I am still convinced that what I had then was "the good life." As I got a little older and heard the phrase, I assumed it meant a lot of money, a big house, a new car, fancy clothes and the ability to do whatever I wanted to do. Close, but no cigar.

I heard the phrase not too long ago, and it caused me to stop and think about what it meant. Just what is "the good life?" Are happiness and the good life the same. I can't answer that for everyone, but, for me, I think it is the same.

I remember an email that I received some time ago (that I

can't find now) that told about a mother and daughter who always wished each other "enough." I find a hint to what "the good life" means to me in that phrase - "I wish you enough." Enough what? In my way of thinking, and I believe it is different for each of us, a good life for me would is having enough:

- money

- beauty

- safety

- nourishment

- friendship

- knowledge/wisdom

- freedom

- challenge

- love

I don't know whether to put pain and heartache on the list. I think they, like salt, are needed to flavor the good life with understanding, compassion, and generosity. In my opinion, they are needed to build character but for some, they are more destructive than constructive, so I'll leave them off.

After I made a list, I looked at it again. (I know this is not an exhaustive, all-encompassing list. It is a list that simply works for me. And my lists have a way of changing over time as I'm sure they do for most list makers). This time I asked myself, which of these things can be left off the list and still allow me to have "the good life?" What can I do without and still be happy?

As I went through the list one item at a time, I discovered that I could leave everything off the list except three things:

1. Nourishment. Food and water are essential for existence. However, expensive "caviar and champagne" are not requisites of life or even "the good life" - nourishment is required, and it doesn't need to be gourmet for survival or happiness.

2. Freedom. I wonder if I hadn't known freedom all my life would I be keenly aware of its absence? If I didn't know the greatness of freedom of both choice and action would I be able to be truly happy without it? I can't answer that. I know that when I've been confined to bed or the house because of illness, my life felt cramped and limited. I hope I never need to discover the answer. For me the good life requires freedom.

3. Love. Love is the sine qua non of happiness or "the good life" for me. Without it, nothing else satisfies, and with it,

nothing else matters. Love is where "it's at." Love. Think about it.

There is one last thing. It is like the ribbon on the package that ties it all together. Appreciation. If I have "more than enough" of everything on my list but don't appreciate any of it, I probably will never know "the good life."

Nourishment, freedom, and love are the big three for me. Add on appreciation and life becomes quite glorious.

I wish you "enough," and that includes an appreciation of everything you have and are.

Have a great day. Have a good life.

The Good Life

If the good life is about having things, how is it that so many people who have so many things have lives that lack so much satisfaction and meaning? I am not saying that having money is not a good thing, quite the contrary. We all need financial security. We need to know that we can provide for our families and be free of the pressure of struggling to make ends meet. We all want to live a comfortable life. But where is the point of no return?

"Not everything that can be counted counts, and not everything that counts can be counted."

Albert Einstein (1879 - 1955), (attributed)

The Worldwide Institute in its 2004 State of the World report explains:

Societies focused on well-being involved more interaction with family, friends, and neighbors, a more direct experience of nature, and more attention to finding fulfillment and creative expression than in accumulating goods. They emphasize lifestyles that avoid abusing your health, other people, or the natural world. In short, they yield a deeper sense of satisfaction with life than many people report experiencing today.

What provides for a satisfying life? In recent years, psychologists studying measures of life satisfaction have largely confirmed the adage that money can't buy happiness- at least not for people who are already affluent. The disconnection between money and happiness in wealthy countries is perhaps most clearly illustrated when growth in income in industrial countries is plotted against levels of happiness. In the United States, for example, the average person's income more than doubled between 1957 and 2002, yet the share of people reporting themselves to be "very happy" over that period remained static.

So if growth in income has not made people happier than obviously, they are not living the good life. To clarify what the good life is, I do an exercise with clients that involves seeing themselves at some distant point in the future where they are finally who they want to be; they have what they want to have and are deeply satisfied and happy. In other words, they have achieved 'Good Life.'

Nearly one hundred percent of the time; without fail, clients do not have visions of extreme wealth. They don't talk about wealth at all, at least not in terms of money or possessions. They do not talk about living in a house with every known convenience and luxury. They do talk about a home located in a beautiful setting, perhaps by the ocean or on a lake in the mountains. There is always talk about a place that gives them a feeling of peace and serenity...a place they were meant to be.

They never discuss possessions...ever. No talk of cars, televisions or fancy clothes. It just never comes up. They may mention that they are free to travel, but certainly, they do not say, first class.

They describe themselves as a person who no longer fights feelings of depression, dissatisfaction or dissonance in their lives. They speak of a feeling of acceptance of what is. There is love in their lives although they don't necessarily mention a specific mate. Just love. There is a discussion of deep wisdom accumulated over the years. There is also talk of being surrounded by the people who they hold dear.

Often, if they have children, they will say that they are happy that they have been able to help their kids but more often is the description of children who have grown into responsible, loving and fulfilled human beings. They describe with pride children who are contributors to the world. I hear about pets in the house and perhaps grandchildren. These are folks who have discovered what truly has meaning for them and what they value.

"Happiness is that state of consciousness which proceeds from the achievement of one's values."

Ayn Rand (1905 - 1982)

Values. What are the things to which you attach value? What is important to you? If you had to create a list of the top five things that you value, what would they be? Would it be money, possessions, power, stature, and authority? Would it be love, family, integrity, freedom, and compassion? Or a combination?

"Try not to become a man of success but rather to become a man of value."

Albert Einstein (1879 - 1955)

We have all heard the adage about what the epitaph on our

tombstone will say or not say. Will it say that she had a powerful job, she flew first class, that she had a Mercedes-Benz and wore only couture? More often you will read on a tombstone that she was a loving Mother and Wife, a charitable person and an outstanding member of the community. Think about how you would like to be remembered? What would you like to hear people say about you at your funeral or memorial? Will it be on how much money you made or how much you consumed? Doubtful.

I remember the funeral of a very dear friend who died suddenly while he was still in his fifties. The Rabbi said that all we have in the end is our good name. Who we were, how we lived, how we loved, our empathy and compassion, service to the world we lived in and the legacy we left to our children and their children.

My take on the good life, at least for me, involves the following: I want to be a person who possesses a deep appreciation for everything that I have: to be grateful. I want to be able to live without the fear of not being able to take care of my kids and myself, and yes, I do want to live well. Living well for me is a lovely home in nature; it is free to travel; it can help my kids get a good start in their adult lives; it has enough money to be able to take good care of myself and also to be charitable. I want to have a life that is filled with meaning, with a deep connection to the world around me.

What is your Good Life? Take the time now to give thought to the life that you want to live, the life that you would describe as the Good Life. Make certain that it is aligned with your values and your passions and to so you must connect with your values and passions. What are they? Think long and hard about what brings you real joy and fulfillment. Remember those times in your life when you were the happiest...what resonated for you in those moments? Consider how you want to be remembered, how you want to look in your children's eyes. What traits do you admire in others and how can you adopt some of those traits? What have been peak experiences in your life and what was it about those experiences that made them so special?

These are the kind of questions that beg our attention. These are the questions that will ultimately lead us to the Good Life. Not the $14,000 dessert but a life well lived with meaning, love, comfort, joy, and fulfillment.

You can live a life that truly works, and you can achieve peak performance in all areas of your life. You can not only survive life's unexpected changes and transitions but also thrive. Powerful change is possible. You are fully capable of creating a life that you choose. Life Coaching is a proven, powerful, one-on-one professional relationship that promises to improve the quality of your life! Learn how to create positive change in your life.

Choose to Live a Better Life

Some people seem to be lucky. They are always in the right place at the right time. Positive opportunities forever seem to come their way. Are they simply lucky or do they have a different approach to life?

Making the decision and choosing to live a better life gives us the power to improve our lives.

- Being receptive to life elevates the quality of life we live: Using all our senses is important. Sound, smell, taste, sight, and touch are often taken for granted. But when we meet someone who is impaired in some way we see how heightened their other senses have become to compensate for the deficit. Become more aware of the value of adding color, texture, fragrance, music and different flavors to our lives. The more we use our senses, the more engaged in life we become.

- Appreciation for what we have is important: Hearing another person's bad news, hearing of disasters are unfortunate ways of us becoming more appreciative of our good fortune. Taking the time to value friends, family, where we live and work, our quality of life, the freedoms that we have are ways to remind ourselves of our good fortune and motivate us to live more fully.

- Respond rather than react: When we are involved in a difficult situation, it is important to pay attention, listen and gain all the facts. This enables us to appreciate another person's point of view before we react and maybe say something inappropriate. We exercise more control in our choices and behavior.

- Take better care of ourselves: Value our good health and invest in it by paying attention to a healthy, balanced diet, exercise, the importance of taking breaks and becoming aware of our stress levels. Having a quiet time where we turn everything off on occasion is a valuable way to de-stress. Turning off the phone, computer, TV and just being silent is healthy from time to time. Spending some time in nature is a good way to unwind. Finding a work/life balance is important.

- Be aware of negative self-talk: We are often harsher with ourselves than we would ever be to another person. Berating ourselves for an accident or a mistake is unnecessary. Would we be so tough on someone else? Being a little kinder and more appreciative of ourselves and the pressures we are under often makes for an improved state of mind.

- Choose to do something really enjoyable: Busy people often struggle to find enough time for family, friends and other obligations, but having some 'me' time is also important in life. Even if it is a thirty-minute swim, a leisurely bath or taking a walk on the beach doing something for yourself is important.

When we decide to take control of our choices and establish positive ways to look after ourselves we become happier, healthier and more relaxed. The people around us benefit from this.

Changing Your Attitude to Live a Better Life

Changing your attitude to live a better life is a matter of making the decision right now to change your attitude. I know it sounds like I am talking in circles. But, what it comes down to, are you deciding to change your attitude about your life. You need to obtain a positive attitude to get what you want in life,

A little story-

I have seen several friends of mine become success stories in life. And I have seen several friends, obtain nothing that they have wanted in this life. What I noticed, and now apply to my life, is a better attitude. One friend had her husband leave her six weeks after she had her first baby. He left her for another woman. She became very negative and bitter. It seemed like she would never learn from her life experiences, and do the right thing.

After about five years, I noticed her life-changing. Her life changed for the better. Do you know what she did? She changed her attitude. She learned from her mistakes and moved on from being bitter and twisted to happy, confident, and carefree. I soon became in awe of my friend. I admit, I also became jealous of her new life. But after thinking about it, I realized, that I deserved to be happy too.

Cheerleading 101! *A fucking Men*

This is where you can make you're positive, life-changing events to live a better life. Make the decision, and stick by it. Tell yourself every day, you can do it. Be your cheerleader! Get up every morning, look in the mirror and tell yourself you can do it. Tell yourself you are wonderful. Play uplifting cheerleading music while telling yourself you are a good person that deserves only the best in life.

Get rid of all negativity!

Tell your negative thoughts to go away. Replace them with

positive thoughts. This is the process you will go through to change your attitude, thus living a better life. Believe in yourself.

The Devil made me do it!

Now, it is said, the Devil is the one thing in your life that is responsible for making you do and think negative thoughts. Get rid of the Devil in your life. Replace him with God. Start going to church. Pray every day. This will help you to become a more positive person. It is a proven fact going to church once a week, helps make you feel more positive about your life. Goodness and positive thoughts will soon replace the negative ones, and you will be on your way to a more positive life.

You can do it! I come from a long line of negative thinking, worriers. If I can change my attitude, make it positive and live a better life, you can too.

Live A Better Life - With Healthy Eating and Healthy Relationships

To live a better life is the desire and dream of most but many just can't seem to find the right balance to achieve their goal. There are two essentials in life, eating, and relationships, where we have some control in our quest to live a better life.

Here are some basic tips for both.

Tips to Live A Better Life With Healthy Eating

There is so much information and advice available, some of which is contradictory, that it's hard to figure out what to do. Most people want to live a better life and feel if they could just lose a few pounds or outfit sizes, life will be better.

The main goal for healthy eating should be for you to feel good about yourself and avoid health problems such as heart disease, diabetes, strokes, arthritis, and cancer, all of which have been associated with being overweight.

Make Better Health and Not Weight Loss the Goal

Eat healthier foods, and you will begin to feel better about yourself and your life. If you make better food choices, i.e., eating more fruits, vegetables, and whole grains, your body will feel better, and you will feel better as well. Find ways to add more fruits and vegetables by adding fresh fruit to meals, i.e., adding fruit to cereals or salads.

Most folks also choose to eat lean meats and include fish and more beans in their daily diets as they seek to live a better life.

If you can reduce the amount of sugar, you consume it will help you succeed in eating healthier. Although sweets have great taste, they have lots of calories and very little nutritional value.

Tips To Live A Better Life With Healthier Relationships

Life is so much easier and better when relationships with spouses or significant others are right. It just makes it easier to get through the day when you don't worry about having stressful conversations with someone because of a broken relationship.

A great way to live a better life is to surround yourself with people who love and respect you and you feel the same way about them.

If you are in a relationship that is frustrating and causing you to lay awake at night or pull your hair out, then fix it before your blood pressure gets out of hand and leads to some other medical complications.

Generally, relationships are strained because of a broken promise or commitment and pride and ego get in the way of forgiveness and restoration.

I would suggest you figure out why your relationship is strained, do your part to repair the broken relationship and work toward forgiving or if you screwed up being forgiven.

If you aren't enjoying your life right now, then you should take steps to learn how to more completely enjoy your life.

There are so many ways to make this happen, but some of the best ways are the simplest. Read on below for the specifics of how to do it.

Tips for a Better Life:

1. Enjoy what you do on your own time: When you are off the clock, don't be distracted by the calls to work even more when you don't have to.

When you are not at work, you shouldn't be thinking about work. It is a simple rule to keep yourself sane and stress-free. Instead, do something that you enjoy for whatever small amount of free time you may have for yourself.

2. Get rid of stuff you don't need: There are a lot of things you don't need lying around your home, and the odds are good that there is someone who would love to use it.

Clear up all that used space in your home and give someone else the opportunity to use all that stuff you no longer have any use for. It is the right thing to do.

3. Take some time for thought: You can just relax and meditate for a while, and all your troubles will float away like so many clouds. It is just the thing to dissolve stress in your life.

Whether you set aside a half hour or just a couple of minutes, this is valuable time separate from the "free time" you set aside. This is the time for quiet reflection.

You don't have to follow all of these tips, and you can come up with some of your own. But these are great starting points to regaining perspective in this wild and confusing world. You can realign your whole way of life to these things and gain a sense of peace and perseverance that will lead to a better life.

Emotional Intelligence - 4 Techniques to Help You Live A Better Life!

The idea of emotional intelligence is a fairly new one to the realm of education and learning processes. Emotional intelligence, when recognized and applied can turn your world around. In olden days, psychologists declared that IQ levels were the only factor that determined a person's success or failure for that matter, in life. However, studies on emotional intelligence tell us that emotions play as important a part, if not greater than IQ levels in your success or failure.

Emotional intelligence encourages us to recognize the emotional states of mind of others around us, and our own as well. When tapped to perfection, this can help us relate better with other people as well as with our selves. This increases success levels by miles.

A person who lacks emotional intelligence finds himself with an empty feeling and resorts to various courses and counselors to help him cope with his emptiness. However, a course or book material can only give you so much teaching. Life itself is the greatest teacher, and while some have an inborn talent to cope well with life and with people, others can focus their attention on these issues to live a more successful life. This article deals with some of the ways you can increase your emotional intelligence levels. This, of course, will help you deal better with your self as well as with those around you.

1) Emotional Literacy - Like everything else you recognize, you need to give a name to every emotion that you can feel. This helps you recognize them even better and thereby helps you control them as well. You'd be surprised by the effects this can have on your state of mind.

2) Use Emotional Energy - Everybody feels angry at times; anger is a common emotion. Rather than try and suppress your anger, find ways to release it productively. Anger produces energy, and this can be used positively or negatively that-s up to you. Never feed the anger, burn it up doing something useful.

3) Be selective with people - when you relate with the right people your mind will remain in a healthy state. If you go around with people, who do not care about other people's emotions some of that could rub off on you. People who do not care about their own emotions can never care about your emotions.

4) Do not blame other people for your state of mind. True, some people are good at getting you down, but your emotional state is finally under your control and if it isn't it should get that way. If you let people run your life, you will never have a life that you can be proud of.

CHAPTER 2: A POSITIVE MINDSET AIDS A BETTER LIFE

What Is Positive Thinking or a Positive Mindset?

Simply, positive thinking is the opposite of negative thinking. Positive thinking might take place in your mind, when you feel happy or when you have achieved something you have wanted to achieve for a while. It's a little voice in your head (the one that's reading these words) that can put us in a more positive frame of mind on a day-to-day basis as we go about our lives.

Positive thinking is also one way a person can experience the feelings of positive emotions such as joy, happiness, excitement.

It may also put a smile on our faces and a bounce in our step, and make us look forward to things more.

Whether one has positive thoughts or negative thoughts, our minds are occupied with thoughts and depending on some factors, for some, positive thinking occurs more often than for others. But the great thing is that positive thinking is a skill that can be taught, learned, practiced and mastered such as you would be taught sports, practice music, learn a new language or master a subject.

Positive thinking can also become a Mind Set which is the next level of just having positive thoughts from time to time. A Positive Mind Set is such that the majority of your thoughts will be positive. And again for some people, the opposite may be true, but through proven steps, tools and practice, anyone can reprogram their mind to counteract negative thoughts and a negative mindset.

Why positive thinking?

Positive thinking is valuable to us in many ways. For example, if you're competing in a cross country or marathon event at a sports day, and you're running and running, feeling like your legs are going to collapse under you and your stitch will kill you,... you feel weak, muscles are melting, your lungs feel like they're going to burst and every step is agony. As many top sports people do, they will use positive thinking to push through, not just to get over the finishing line, but to win. A positive mindset is also referred to as a "Winner's Mind Set."

Who wouldn't want that?

And as we have established, positive thinking is the opposite of negative thinking. Negative thinking is the other voice or even other voices in our heads that might tell us we are stupid when we make mistakes or fail at something.

Negative thinking can mentally paralyze some people too and stop us from asking for what we want in our lives. For others, it might make them worry about things that may or may not happen.

With a positive mindset, you end up making better decisions, feel good and generally function better in life.

Positive thinking fuels positive energy which is much higher and lighter energy than negative thinking and negative energy which is heavier and brings you down.

Imagine you are invited to go to a party or an event and you think negative thoughts such as,

"I won't go; no one will like me; I hate those people anyway."

Do you think you would be getting off to a good start to make new friends let alone a good impression? You probably will end up not even going.

What if you went into it thinking?

"How fun, new outfit!! I'll wear my new shoes!! All these new people I can get to know (or get to know me) I'm going to have so much fun!"

Which mindset do you think is going to end up having more energy and who do you think will go, stay and meet new friends at the party?

Positive thinking is not... about lying to yourself or being fake. It's important to be realistic and truthful. Your brain will know if you aren't authentic.

To begin thinking positive and living a life from a positive mindset, we have to start noticing positive things that occur all day long. This is being "conscious."

Being conscious is being aware of the thoughts you have, both positive and negative. It is also about noticing what's going on around you and how you internally react to these things and then translate and digest them into being positive or negative.

So to develop your positive thinking skills, beginning with being conscious is important. This is so you can differentiate between negative and positive thoughts as they occur.

A Positive Mindset - A Happier Life

No-one ever said that life is easy. Indeed, the peaks and troughs of life are what make the world go round. Peaks are great but experiencing the troughs need not be such a bad thing either. The important factor is how you deal with them, and this is likely to be much easier if you approach them with a positive mindset.

A positive mindset is very important for many reasons. Positive thinking has been shown to enhance the quality and productivity of life. When we are in a positive frame of mind we feel better, perform better, are healthier and are more productive. We are happier and better equipped to deal with all life throws at us.

Ongoing benefits of a positive attitude include better mental and physical health. This is due to the positive hormones that boost the immune system. We will feel happier and stronger and thus, are likely to be more successful in life.

The reverse is also true. A negative mindset can cause depression. When we are feeling low, we are far more susceptible to contracting the disease and suffering from other mental health issues. It can also cause our relationships to deteriorate, affect our ability to think rationally and our productivity can all but grind to a halt. To sum up, a negative frame of mind should be avoided at all costs. Of course, it is only natural for us to feel low or unhappy at various times in our lives, but it is how we deal with those feelings that are most important.

A positive mindset will give you a 'can do' attitude and you are more likely to see a challenge rather than a problem and to see an opportunity rather than an obstacle. For example, the reason entrepreneurs are so successful is that they can spot opportunities for expansion in areas where others see a downturn. The positive mindset of successful entrepreneurs means that opportunities become realities because they have had the foresight, drive, and motivation to make their dreams come true.

Having a positive mindset is a huge personal asset, but the main challenge for most people is in developing the right mindset in the first place.

The following will help you on your path to a more positive attitude and a happier life:

1. Use only positive words, whenever you think "I can't" replace it with "I can." Don't just think it, say it out loud

2. Train your mind to focus on the good things you have in life, not the bad.

3. Dreading an occasion, conversation or event? Think positively and visualize the best outcome rather than the worst.

4. Whenever negative thoughts creep into your mind; challenge them and replace them with positives. Some people can appear to have a naturally happier disposition than others but, no matter how pessimistic you are, that can

be achieved with a more positive mindset and is something open to anyone prepared to take the necessary steps to attain it.

Why Do You Need a Positive Attitude to Go Through Life?

When people talk about the importance of having a positive attitude, the burning question in your head could be: Why? I am perfectly fine the way I am; why change my attitude? While there is nothing wrong with the way you are but perhaps you could lead a better quality of life in terms of health and happiness, if you consciously developed a more positive outlook towards life. But how do you do this? Here are some guidelines:

Developing a positive attitude starts with how you feel about yourself. If you are confident and self-assured, your positive spirit can be infectious, and you would end up spreading confidence and cheer all around.

A negative feeling about yourself, on the other hand, would also be communicated to others. You not only feel bad about the way you are, but you also make others feel bad about you too.

Though difficult in today's time of war and increased hatred around us, try to focus more on positive things in life. Read and watch things which have a positive impact on your mind.

For beginners who are just learning how to develop a positive state of mind, the recommended procedure is to start with reading funny books, watching humorous movies, spending more time with children, laughing and being happy. All these activities push you more towards positivism.

Your positive attitude can be a great source of joy and relief for people around you. You do not have to sermonize to them or give them free advice; you simply exude that warmth and comfort to distressed people by sitting close to them.

All of us know that life perhaps is tilted more towards negative incidents and people than positive situations. Despite your environment, if you try sincerely, you can still overcome these negativisms around you and develop a positive attitude, to lead a more fruitful, happier and more meaningful existence.

How to Use Positive Thinking to Change Your Life

Working with energy and the power of the mind is the most powerful way to make changes in your life. The principle of the Law of Attraction is based on this and is being used by people from all over the world. It is a simple concept; however, making this principle work for you can be harder than it seems.

Using Positive Thoughts to Create Change

Positive thinking does work. You will attract back to, you the kind of energy that you put out. For example, if you are thinking angry thoughts, then you will attract anger back to you. Once this concept is understood, you can begin to control your daily experiences by controlling what thoughts go through your head and what energy you are putting out there.

Believe it or not, you are using this principle every single day. The problem comes in when you realize you are not necessarily attracting all of the things that you want which could mean you are not projecting the right kind of energy or thinking positive thoughts.

Not as easy as it Seems

Thoughts become very habitual, and it is not always so easy to change them. You may not even be aware of the thoughts you are thinking half the time. Often when people begin trying to implement positive thinking into their life, there are times when they feel like a failure. However, I have learned that it is important to stick with it. Once you become fully aware of your thoughts and your energy, you will become better and better at learning to control it and work with it.

It Takes a Lot of Practice

Using positive thinking to your benefit does take a lot of practice. It is not just a quick fix as many would like you to believe. It is a way of life and consequently takes a lifetime of continuous practice.

A Little Help Along the Way

There are several ways to improve your thinking habits and energy. The most popular, way is to simply make a point of being aware of every thought that goes through your head.

Meditation practice is another great way to incorporate positive energy into your life. Binaural beats are a type of brainwave audio that is also extremely helpful and have made a big difference for me. By incorporating these practices into your habits and your life, you will create a new reality that just keeps improving as you get better and better at projecting positive and beneficial energy.

It can be very rewarding to work with your energy and to realize how much control you have over your own life. I would only suggest that you be patient with yourself and if you need a little help along the way... get it.

Essential Tools for Positive Thinking and a Positive Mindset

Here are some proven tools that you can apply and practice daily to begin developing a positive mindset.

First, you need to begin by allocating time for it in your life as if it were a part of your routine such as brushing your teeth.

Journaling - Two Parts

Part one: Begin with a gratitude journal. To do this, you can either use a notebook and pen, laptop, iPhone (smartphone) or iPad.

Start with the date. Then either write the following instruction down and begin your list or just go ahead and begin your list.

Part two: Checking in with how you feel.

This next part of developing a positive mindset is to record how you feel throughout the day. Set a reminder for yourself for the following times:

- Morning

- Mid-Morning

- Lunchtime

- Mid Afternoon

- Evening

- Late evening

Ask yourself how you feel and write down one emotion or feeling (of course it can be more!).

(Hint: Make a list of emotions on a small piece of paper and keep it in your wallet or purse. This will help you to easily identify your feelings and emotions quickly if this is not something you are used to.)

- Happy

- Joyful

- Tired

- Sad

- Melancholy

- Excited

- Worried

- Nervous

- Anxious

- Worry Time

Positive thinking is not about a land of pretense and fake smiles. Part of developing a positive mindset is to also acknowledge the things that worry us. Things like issues that come up with studies, exams, relationships, arguments, changes at home or school, the future and even the past.

It is important to not be in denial; otherwise, we might find ourselves in situations that we could have prevented by allocating "worry time" in our day.

And, the benefit is that if we can be proactive about issues that come up calmly, we end up making better decisions; better judgments and come up with better ideas and solutions than if we are feeling emotional and right in the middle of it all, all day long.

By allocating the fixed amount of time, such as 15 minutes, we allow ourselves to be free from stewing over those things all day long. This then allows us to enjoy all the rest of the good moments that occur throughout the day.

To do this:

Make a list of the things that are worrying you.

Allocate and spend 15 minutes making a list of your worries and coming up with possible solutions.

Many problems cannot be solved all at once, so don't worry that you haven't solved them in the time allocated. But, by spending just 15 minutes a day and focussing on coming up with solutions, you are putting your time and energy to much better use, than by worrying all day long. Inch by inch you're getting closer and closer to the solution. You get back in charge again.

Problem-solving steps:

- Look for the cause of the problem

- Brainstorm possible solutions (free flow of ideas)

- Choose the best solution

- Plan to or implement the solution

Worry time tips:

Keep it separate from your gratitude journal, so just create another word document or note or if you have a notebook, write it in another one or at least in the back of your gratitude journal

In the day if we recognize an existing problem that is worrying us and cannot solve it right then and there, allocate it to worry time.

If it is a new problem, make a note and again, if you cannot deal with it then and there, allocate it to worry time.

If we come up with an idea to solve the worry in the day, also make a note and delegate this to your worry time slot.

After you have spent your 15 minutes of worry time, open your gratitude journal and read over the things you have written. You can repeat these in your mind like a personal mantra. What this is doing, is blocking out all thought except for the thoughts of the things we are happy about.

NB. Some problems will not be solvable. At the moment you realize the problem cannot be solved, is the moment they become someone else's problem and can be taken off your list!

Meditation

Meditation, mentioned before, is most effective and beneficial when it's done as often as possible.

Daily practice (is the key!).

Meditation is a mental discipline and helps us to become more conscious. There are different types of meditations that have different outcomes, and we can incorporate positive thoughts into a meditation session using mantras. Mantras are true positive statements that are repeated in our minds and sometimes said out loud to replace any negative thoughts.

Muscle relaxation exercises

Muscle relaxation exercises train us to better recognize when our bodies might be reacting to a stressful or upsetting situation which prevents us from being fully relaxed and in control of our thoughts and therefore preventing us from creating positive thoughts too.

Stress Management diary

This is a bit like the worry time and useful for those of you who are feeling stressed out. A stress management diary allows you to see patterns and if done correctly, can provide you with permanent solutions to things that stress you out.

Affirmations

Affirmations allowed us to consciously empower our minds and reprogram it at a subconscious level (the bank of thoughts and information in our minds we don't use all the time) and replace all those old untrue negative thoughts about ourselves. Affirmations can be used in meditation and developing a positive self-image and are most effective when spoken aloud, are easy to say and rhythmic.

Essential Tips for affirmations: Make sure you use positive words. The key is to state what you do want, not what you don't want. Also, affirmations are only effective when we speak for ourselves as we cannot change others, e.g., "I am at peace with my sister," NOT, "my sister and I don't fight anymore."

The main point is you have a choice - you can change how you feel if you want to.

When you are feeling worried and scared, jealous, stressed, angry, bitter or resentful and can't shake it. Ask yourself this question:

"How do I want to feel?"

I'm sure you'll come up with something different to what you are feeling in those bad times. Then, follow the steps above, and if you practice, sooner than later you will find things that may have affected you in the past are like water of a duck's back.

Developing a positive self-image

This is a skill that tops everything off and is especially important when our bodies begin to change before we know it! When we have a positive self-image, we feel comfortable with who we are and what we are doing in our lives. And although many of us don't know who we are or what we want to do with our lives, what's great about this technique is that it doesn't matter!

To start developing a positive self-image, you start with a 'wish list' of what we would like to be true about ourselves. For example:

"I wish I was slimmer."

Then, in a column next to it you write an affirmation to correspond with the desire.

"My body's natural state is good health. Physical activity comes naturally"

Positive thinking checklist

- Daily journaling

- Daily worry time

- Practice Meditation daily

- Muscle relaxation exercises daily

- Stress Management diary weekly

- Affirmations as needed

- Developing a positive self-image NOW!

CHAPTER 3: GOOD SLEEP FOR A BETTER LIFE

What Is Sleep? Understand the Basics

From a medical point of view, sleep can be understood as a state of mind experiencing reduced levels of consciousness involving temporary inactivity of nearly all voluntary muscles, and a relative suspension of sensory and non-motor activity. In simple terms, sleep is an impermanent physical and mental state of the mind during which most of the external stimuli are blocked from the senses, and the individual stops responding to the environment. There are different types of "sleep" depending upon the intensity and manifestation of sleeping criteria. The ability of the person to "awake," or come out from the transitory partial inactive state of mind depends upon several factors, and these factors vary from person-to-person. Even though it can't be proved on a conclusive basis, medical experts believe the basic purpose of sleep is to create a state of inertness in the human body, during which the body can repair itself and regulate the metabolism to improve its functioning, and the state of inertness helps save the energy which is utilized for the rejuvenation process.

Repair theory

As per this theory, during the "awake" period, the body is physically and mentally responding to the various activities associated with our daily activities, and this consumes large amounts of energy. The energy utilized is depleted from the energy reserves stored in various parts of the body. The replenishment and body repair activities can occur effectively when the body is undergoing a state of rest - when no extra energy is utilized for any physical processes or activities. The sleep period ensures all the resources in the body are utilized in an optimum manner for the maintenance and upkeep of the various metabolic processes occurring in our body that keep us alive.

Adaptive theory

According to this theory, sleep is a naturally evolved phenomenon that humans and animals adapted to for their survival. Sleeping helps in preserving energy and prevents exposure to dangers and predators.

How "sleep" works?

As far as the process of sleeping is concerned, scientists believe that our metabolism has two processes:

• The sleep-wake process

• Circadian biological clock or Circadian rhythm Which regulate our sleep. Both the processes function in tandem, and create the "sleep cycle" because of which we tend to feel sleepy at night, and remain awake during the day. The processes regulate our sleep cycle, which scientists believe is essential for body repair and sustenance. The Circadian biological clock can be understood as a 24-hour condition during which the body rhythm is affected by sunlight. The presence and absence of sunlight control the secretion of certain essential hormones in the body. The melatonin hormone (N-acetyl-5-methoxytryptamine) is secreted in the absence of sunlight, generally at night, and is primarily responsible for regulating the body temperature. The cycle needs to be in accord with the physical state of the individual and the metabolic functioning of the body.

Circadian rhythm or the "sleep cycle."

Circadian rhythm is an approximately 24-hour cycle associated with the biochemical, physiological, and behavioral processes. The term "circadian" is derived from the Latin word "circa" which means "around," and "Diem" or "dies" which means "day." Therefore, the term means "approximately one day." The rhythm is generated by a metabolic activity which functions as an internal body clock, and which is synchronized with the "light-dark" cycles as well as the changes taking place in the subject's environment.

Stages of sleep

The sleep process consists of two main stages which keep on repeating in a cycle of 90 to 110 minutes during the entire sleeping activity. The two stages are:

• REM (Rapid Eye Movement)

• Non-REM (Non - Rapid Eye Movement, which is further classified into four substages)

REM sleep

The Rapid Eye Movement (REM) stage of sleep is characterized by a rapid movement of the eyes, in addition to a low muscle tone, and partial paralysis of all voluntary muscles. In the case of humans, this type of sleep occupies between 20% to 25% of the total sleep duration - approximately 90 to 120 minutes. Typically, about four to five cycles occur during normal REM sleep. The duration of the cycle is short at the beginning of the sleep and starts extending towards the end. The exact duration of REM sleep required can't be ascertained since the sleep cycle varies from individual to individual as per the body's metabolic requirements. In the case of newborn babies, the REM stage consists of around 80% of the total sleeping time. REM sleep is also affected by the aging process. During the REM stage, no dominate brain waves are emitted as per polysomnogram findings. The first REM cycle usually begins approximately 70 to 90 minutes after the sleeping process commences, i.e., after falling asleep. During the REM stage, even though the subject is not responsive to any strong external stimuli, the brain remains active, and as per polysomnogram tests, the degree of activity is considerably more as compared to the "awake" stage. The REM stage is also associated with the "dreaming" phenomenon, and when the process occurs, the frequency of REM, i.e., the movement of eyes increases significantly. Typically, depending upon the intensity of the dreaming activity, the blood pressure too is affected and can increase marginally or significantly.

Non-REM sleep

The Non-REM sleep stage is characterized by an absence of rapid eye movement, a decrease in the metabolic activity, a reduction in the breathing and heart rates, and generally a substantial decrease amounting to almost an absence of dreaming activity. Unlike the REM stage, voluntary muscles do not experience a partial paralysis in this stage. The non-rem stage is composed of four sub stages - stage 1 associated with light sleep, stage 2 by true sleep, and stages 3 and 4 with deep sleep. In human adults, Non-REM sleep comprises about 75% to 80% of the total sleeping time. The stages are as follows:

Stage 1: Light sleep

During the "awake" stage, the brain emits alpha waves having a frequency between 8 to 13 Hz. On the onset of the first stage of Non-REM sleep, the brain undergoes a gradual transition during which the intensity of the waves emitted starts decreasing, and reaches between 4 to 7 Hz characterized by the theta waves. This stage may involve slow eye movement, twitches, and even "hypnic jerks" commonly referred to as "sleep start" or "night start" during which the subject awakens suddenly just when he or she is about to fall asleep. The voluntary muscles and metabolic activities start slowing down. The individual can be easily awakened during this stage of sleep.

Stage 2: True sleep

Generally within 10 to 15 minutes of the first stage of light sleep, the second stage of true sleep sets in which lasts approximately between 20 to 25 minutes. This second stage of Non-REM sleep is characterized by "sleep spindles" ranging from 11 to 16 Hz during which the brain inhibits various processes to keep the subject in a tranquil state, and the K-complex which suppresses cortical arousal to prevent any external stimuli from signaling danger and aid sleep-based memory consolidation. During this stage, no eye movements occur, and the breathing pattern, as well as the heart rate, slows down. This stage comprises about 45% to 55% of the total sleep consumed by adults.

Stages 3 and 4: Deep sleep

During the third stage of Non-REM sleep, the brain starts emitting delta waves having a high amplitude (75 µV) and low-frequency (0.5 to 2 Hz). The breathing and heart rates are at their lowest. Parasomnias - a category of sleep disorders associated with abnormal and unnatural body movements, abnormal behavior pattern, uncontrolled emotions, and abnormal perceptions generally occur during this stage. Sleeping disorders such as night terrors, sleepwalking, nocturnal enuresis (bedwetting), and somniloquy (talking aloud in one's sleep) are also associated with this stage. The fourth stage of Non-REM sleep is associated with rhythmic breathing and restricted muscle activity.

Dreams

From a scientific point of view, there is no fixed definition of "dreaming." A dream can be interpreted as a succession of images, sounds, and emotions that the human mind experiences during the sleeping process. The basic purpose and manifestation of the dreaming phenomenon are still not clearly understood, and scientists have several hypotheses which try to explain the process. However, it is commonly believed amongst scientists that dreams are a result of certain psychological, or neuropsychological activities occurring in a certain portion of the brain. Dreams are associated with the psychological aspect of the brain - the non-tangible part (mind), and not the tangible part (brain). It's important to differentiate between the two. During the lifetime, it is believed a human being spends approximately six years dreaming, which comes to around two hours daily as an average if we are to consider the average life span of a person. It is still unknown exactly how and why dreams originate, and whether there is a single origin, or multiple portions of the brain are involved.

Difference between REM and Non-REM sleep dreams

There is a subtle difference between the dreams occurring during the REM and Non-REM stages of sleep. Dreams occurring during the Non-REM stage are brief and fragmentary, do not have any lasting impression on the individual, and they are easily forgotten. In this particular stage, the individual is less likely to experience any lucid and clear visual images resulting out of the dreaming process. During the REM dream stage, a portion of the brain called "pons" shuts off all chemical signals associated with voluntary muscles functioning to the spinal cord. This causes temporary paralysis, and the body becomes incapable of any voluntary movements. The REM sleep signal originates from the pons. This is a natural defense mechanism which prevents the person from harming himself or herself during sleep, since the dreams occurring during the REM stage of sleep can seem to be real and life-like, and this can cause the subject to respond physically in accordance to the particular dream pattern. It is believed pons secretes acetylcholine, a chemical compound that acts as a neurotransmitter, during the REM stage which is transmitted to different parts of the forebrain. This causes cholinergic activation within the affected tissue areas. This is what causes the "dream" phenomenon.

High Quality Sleep Is Critical for Good Health

Most people believe that all sleep is the same, as long as you sleep. This is not true. There are, in fact, two types of sleep: high quality and poor quality. And some people enjoy high-quality sleep night after night, while others rarely encounter it. Poor quality sleep can easily be seen by looking at the brain waves of people while they are sleeping. These waves are fragmented in places and are generally quite different from the waves around them.

Poor quality sleep leaves you feeling sluggish, drained, out-of-sorts and sleepy during the day. Indeed, if you feel this way, it's a good indication your sleep is of poor quality. High quality sleep, on the other hand:

- Restores and revitalizes your body and mind.

- Helps you avoid depression and anxiety.

- Decreases your risk of heart and cardiovascular disease.

- Revitalizes your immune system.

- Improves your concentration and memory during the day.

Indeed, you should be able to feel many of these things during the following day, and if you don't, it may mean that you are experiencing poor quality sleep.

Although it might seem that your body is inactive while you are sleeping, this is not true. Important changes are going on. They include:

- Your heart rate and blood pressure decrease.

- Your breathing rate decreases.

- Your body temperature drops slightly.

- Growth hormones are released.

- Cortisol is released (some is also released during the day).

These things are all critical for regenerating your body and getting it ready for the next day. They do not take place as efficiently and smoothly as they should during poor quality sleep. And this is one of the reasons you don't feel fully recharged and ready for the day.

You can see the problem more closely if you look in detail at how sleep occurs. It's not as simple as going to sleep, then waking 8 hours later. Your body undergoes 4 or 5 cycles of about 90 minutes each night. Each of these cycles consists of two stages of light sleep, two stages of deep sleep, and a stage of REM, or dream, sleep. Each of these stages can easily be seen in the waves that your brain gives off during the night. Both the frequency (speed) and amplitude (height) of these waves changes as you sleep. The major change is that they slow down, and their amplitude increases.

The first stages of sleep, referred to as one and two, are light sleep, and they occur soon after you fall asleep. Your brain waves are still relatively rapid, but as you continue sleeping they slow down and you enter stage 3, then stage 4 of what is referred to as deep sleep. It is very difficult to rouse you from a deep sleep. You can spend up to 45 minutes in a deep sleep (young people spend the most time here), but eventually, you re-enter light sleep. And finally, you pass into REM or dream sleep. This is the point where you are closest to being awake, and your brain waves have speeded up considerably. You can dream anywhere from a few minutes to twenty minutes or more; then you go back to stage 2 light sleep, then deep sleep. You go through this cycle 4 or 5 times during the night.

If you are a good sleeper, everything goes smoothly, and you don't wake up. (Actually, almost everyone wakes up for very short periods during the night, but they go back to sleep quickly and don't remember waking.)

The brain waves associated with high-quality sleep are generally uniform within each stage, and the transition from stage to stage is smooth. The brain waves of poor sleepers, on the other hand, have an irregular section in them referred to as fragmentations that are broken-up and irregular. They are, basically, a sudden change from slow regular waves to fast waves that resemble wakefulness. Large numbers of these fragmentations occur over the night. Not all of them wake the person up, so someone with poor quality sleep frequently doesn't realize that he or she is not sleeping soundly.

These fragmentations cause many problems for sleepers, including:

- Not enough deep sleep.

- Not enough REM sleep.

- Broken and irregular cycles.

- Too much light sleep.

Sudden changes in normal body changes at night.

They also tend to make the sleeper toss and turn a lot during the night, and this is also an indication of poor quality sleep. The first two on the above list are very important because deep sleep and REM are the two most important stages of sleep. Deep sleep regenerates your body, and REM sleep appears to regenerate your mind.

What all this boils down to is: if you want the benefits of high-quality sleep, you'll have to get rid of the fragmentation seen in poor quality sleep. How do you do this? Many long and comprehensive lists of what you should do for good sleep exist and I won't try to cover everything; I'll concentrate only on the things that are most critical for eliminating fragmentation and poor quality sleep. They are:

Good sleep patterns begin with changes during the day,

particularly the hour or so before bedtime. During this last hour, you should relax and wind down. It's also important to stick to the same schedule (particularly bed-time) day after day.

If you are properly primed at bedtime a "wave of sleepiness" will occur. Wait for it, if possible.

Tossing and turning causes much of fragmentation, so get as comfortable as possible using a proper pillow, mattress, covers and so on.

Thoroughly relax when you go to bed. Let yourself go! Leave all problems behind.

It is critical once you are in bed to eliminate all "racing thoughts," particularly negative thoughts and thoughts related to work or any problems you might have.

Don't worry about anything. In particular, don't worry if you don't fall asleep fast enough. Enjoy your relaxation. Think of it as fun.

After turning off all thought and enjoying your feeling, try to enlist images of quiet, peaceful places you have enjoyed. Concentrate on them. Visualize them.

Five Basic Rules for Better Sleep

Millions of people have trouble sleeping. It's estimated that ten percent of Americans suffer from insomnia at any given time, and as a result, millions of sleeping pills are consumed every night. There are, however, several things you can do that will significantly improve your sleep, and surprisingly, many of the people who suffer from insomnia never use them. It's well-known that sleep is affected by both physiological (body) and psychological (mind) factors, and both must be addressed if you are to improve your sleep.

The body factors are related to what is called the "body clock." In reality, there are several body clocks. One is related directly to sleep; several others are indirectly related in that they regulate the hormones that your body gives off at night such as melatonin, serotonin, growth hormone and cortisol. A clock also regulates your body temperature throughout the night. Under ideal circumstances, these clocks are all synchronized.

The psychological or mind factors that affect your sleep are your thought, emotions, anxieties, stress and so on. They are usually associated with an overactive mind, and people with insomnia have been shown to have overactive minds; in particular, their minds are cluttered with anxious thoughts that create negative emotions and stresses that don't allow them to sleep. You have to control both your body clock and your thought if you want a good night's sleep. Five rules that will help you do this are as follows:

1. Start by re-setting (or re-aligning) your body clock.

Your body clock is like an ordinary clock in that it has a period of 24 hours, and like ordinary clocks, it can get out of aligning. What does this mean? Your body clock adjusts to your schedule of sleep and wakefulness, and because it knows this schedule, it tells your body when to get ready for bed, and when to rise in the morning. As long as you keep a regular schedule, this clock will operate effectively. But if you stay up late and begin sleeping in, particularly on weekends, your body clock can't adjust properly, and you find you aren't sleeping when you're supposed to be or waking up before you normally do. In short, your body clock has been knocked out of adjustment and needs to be re-set.

Furthermore, your body clock controls your body temperature at night. It allows it to decrease by one or two degrees until about 4: oo A.M. then it begins to rise slowly. About two hours later it gives you a wake-up call. If your bedtime and rise time are irregular, this clock is not sure when to wake you. So you have to re-set it by getting back to a regular schedule.

2. Once your body clock is reset, you have to develop sufficient sleep drive, which in turn creates a sleep "pressure" that puts you to sleep.

You create a sleep drive by creating a "sleep debt." Most people stay awake approximately 16 out of the 24 hours of the day. This means they have an 8-hour sleep debt when they go to bed. If you're having problems sleeping, however, an 8-hour sleep debt may not be enough to put you to sleep quickly. Your sleep debt, which creates your sleep drive, is increased by staying awake and active as long as possible during the day. In particular, make sure you get as much sunlight as possible (it's sunlight that builds up your sleep drive). Also, you should not nap during the day (assuming you have insomnia), and you should make sure you don't sleep in to make up for sleep you may have lost during the night. If you lost some sleep (assuming you don't sleep in) your sleep drive will be greater the next night because you'll have a larger sleep debt. This will create extra "pressure' for you to sleep.

3. Make sure you "prepare" yourself for sleep

Many people are tense and have anxious thoughts throughout the day (mostly because of our fast, high-pressure, society, and they have trouble relaxing before they go to bed. Their mind is in "full gear" all day long, and they are unable to shut it down before they go to bed. It's important, however, to make sure you "let go" before you go to bed. There are usually two types of thoughts in their minds: non-emotional and emotional. Tthe worst are the emotional thoughts, but non-emotional (decisions, planning for the next day) thoughts can also be a problem. It's important to allow for a "cool down" period before you go to bed to get rid of them. This means you should spend at least half-an-hour (or preferably, an hour) relaxing and preparing yourself for sleep. Several of the things you can do during this time is:

- read

- watch TV (make sure it is nonviolent)

- take a warm bath

- meditate

Make sure your mind is "quiet" before you go to bed. Also, you should make sure you are sleepy. If you're not sleepy, wait until you are.

4. Once in bed, don't try to force yourself to sleep

The object, once you are in bed is to allow yourself to go to sleep as quickly as possible. If you are awake for a half-hour or longer, don't fall into the trap of trying to force yourself to sleep. This is, in fact, the worst thing you can do. Think about when you were younger and slept well. Did you go to bed and "try to sleep?" No, sleep just came -- usually with no effort. So don't try to force yourself to sleep -- let it come naturally. This may seem like it is easier said than done. But if your sleep drive is well-primed and you have a good sleep debt, you will sleep. If you're still awake after an hour or so, get up, go to another room and read or meditate until you are sleepy.

5. Quiet your mind

If you are still having problems, you will have to quiet your mind further, and there are a couple of different approaches to this. The first thing is to completely clear your mind -- make it blank. Then think of an enjoyable image: a mountain scene you once saw, an enjoyable day at the beach, or a family gathering. Keep your mind fixed on it. Relax and enjoy it until you fall asleep.

Finally, don't worry if you don't get 7 or 8 hours of sleep. Any sleep you lose will help build up a better sleep drive for the following night. And don't worry if you wake up in the night. Accept it, relax, roll over and go back to sleep.

Starting a Healthy Sleep Routine

Sleep is vital to your health and wellbeing; the average adult needs between seven and eight hours of sleep daily to feel their best. Our work and social responsibilities, however, can cause stress which disrupts our normal sleep schedule and deprives us of the rest we need for optimal health.

If you've been having problems getting to sleep or staying asleep, the following tips can help you to establish a healthy sleep routine that will allow you to stay in better health.

1. Set a regular sleep schedule and stick to it as closely as possible. When you go to sleep and wake at roughly the same time every day, you're working by your natural circadian rhythms. Avoid sleeping late, even when you don't have to go to work. When you oversleep, you're not making up for losing sleep by going to bed later than normal.

2. Avoid using stimulants like caffeine or nicotine close to bedtime. These substances are notorious for keeping people awake; in fact, it's best to avoid using either in the eight hours preceding your usual bedtime. Even though it's a depressant rather than a stimulant, alcohol is also known to disrupt sleep and should also be avoided before going to sleep.

3. Do not have heavy meals or large intakes of liquids before

going to bed. Dinner should be a light meal and be eaten at least two hours before your bedtime. Foods which tend to cause heartburn or stomach upset should not be eaten before bed for obvious reasons. Drinking too much liquid before bed should be avoided to prevent the need to wake up throughout the night to answer nature's call.

4. Get regular exercise. Exercise is great for helping you to maintain body weight and generally stay in shape - and regular exercise also helps you maintain a regular sleep schedule and get deeper, more restful sleep. While exercise is a great thing, exercising right before bedtime is not; this can make it harder to get to sleep. Try to schedule your workouts for the early morning or early evening.

5. Make sure that your bedroom provides a proper environment for sleeping. The place where you sleep should be dark, quiet and comfortable.

6. Relax before bedtime to wind down from your day. Soft music, a warm bath or reading are all good ways to relax and prepare for sleep. If you're having trouble sleeping, try not to get worked up about it - this will only make it harder to sleep. If you can't get to sleep within 20 minutes, get up and try doing something relaxing before returning to bed.

7. Having trouble getting to sleep once in a while is normal, but having trouble falling or staying asleep regularly is not. If

your inability to get to sleep is becoming a problem, see your physician find out if you have a sleep disorder and if so, seek treatment.

If you're having difficulty establishing a healthy sleep routine, try these seven suggestions; they have worked for many. If you have a sleep disorder, then seek treatment as soon as possible - sleep is too important to your health to live with this kind of problem.

7 Tips for Better Sleep

Do you find yourself lying in bed at night tossing and turning or counting backward in the hopes of eventually falling asleep? If you suffer from occasional bouts of insomnia, here are seven sleep aids that can help you sleep with more ease:

1. With the increased awareness of the importance of receiving a good night's sleep, some sleep-friendly pillows are now available for sleep-hungry individuals. Some pillows are specifically designed to help reduce the frequency and intensity of snoring.

Snoring is one of the greatest detractors to a good night's sleep. The new PillowPositive is a special patented cervical pillow. Clinical trials have shown its efficacy in helping reduce snoring. Pillow Positive encourages the user to position their head to avoid positions that leave the airway passages vulnerable to snoring.

Another sleep-friendly pillow is the Nelson Sound Sleeper. The Nelson Sound Sleeper is an ergonomically designed pillow that has built-in speakers that allow relaxing music to be funneled to the user. The Nelson Sound Sleeper is made for the whole body. It supports a healthy inclined position that reflects the body's natural curvature, and which supports the spine. The Nelson Sound Sleeper is designed to support and distribute equally the user's body weight, regardless of what side or sleeping position the sleeper has taken.

2. Aromatherapy sleep aids that will send you off to dreamland sweetly. Although many people scoffed when aromatherapy first caught the public's attention, research shows that essential oils can be quite effective in alleviating all sorts of medical conditions. Lavender has proven to be the most popular choice for inducing sleep.

There are several ways you can use lavender to fall asleep. You can purchase a special aromatherapy diffuser that you can use to expel the aroma in your bedroom before bedtime. You can place a few drops in your hot bath, or you can purchase lavender massage oil and rub it into your skin before nighttime.

Whatever you choose, you will want to remember that essential oils can be surprisingly powerful--a few drops goes a long way. You can also create a small sachet filled with lavender potpourri that you can place in your pillow. Some people have also reported success with the use of jojoba oil, marjoram, and ylang-ylang.

3. White noise machines can be particularly effective if you need to fall asleep during the day, where distractions and noise are more prone to keep you awake. Popular models include the Norelco Natural Sound Selector, the Burltech Ultra Heart, and Sound Soother, and the Marpac line of Sound Conditioners. Most of these white noise machines are outfitted with several modes and sounds from nature that are designed to send you off to sleep.

A simpler way to gain a similar effect is to use a fan on a low setting or to set the radio on the classical music station at a very low volume.

4. Like essential oils, music is another great way to calm the senses and prepare the body for restful sleep. Many musical CDs specifically designed to send you off to sleep are now available. The SleepNowCD, for instance, contains sonic biofeedback that is designed to minimize anxiety and induce

sleep. Another option for insomniacs is the Easy Sleep Tapes for Insomniacs from Hypnosis Concepts. These tapes contain two hypnosis sessions aimed to ease you into a restful sleep.

5. Certain herbs have been proven to induce sleep. Special nighttime or sleepy time teas can be a powerful yet natural method to induce sleep. Chamomile, valerian, and ginger teas are recommended for sleep-seekers. Make sure to drink these hot teas at least an hour before bedtime.

6. If you find yourself experiencing transient insomnia due to travel or temporary stressors, over the counter sleep aids can help you get the rest you need quickly and easily. Over the counter sleep aids is no substitute for natural sleep, and their use should be discontinued as soon as possible. These drugs are designed to provide fast relief from sleeplessness, but they lose their effectiveness if used for too long.

7. With the variety of non-drug sleep aids now available, prescription sleep aids should be avoided, if possible. If you suffer from severe chronic insomnia, visit your doctor to make sure you are not suffering from an underlying disorder or illness. Many sleep aids carry the risk of side effects, and some can even be addictive. Proceed with caution when it comes to prescription sleep aids.

You can search the web for information on treatments to

reverse wrinkles or simply visit our site. Visit our site often, and you'll be well informed when is comes to non-surgical facelifts and effective anti-aging products, medical treatments & body and mind health.

Diet for Sound Sleep

In simple words, it is not good to not have gained proper sleep. Thus one needs to ensure that they eat well so that they can receive proper sleep.

Ever came across people who would go on a diet and found it difficult to sleep in the night? We should eat light meals, those that are not hard to be digested. Avoid intake of meals which are high in calories and make you feel heavy in the chest after consumption.

Drink plenty of water.

Do not have caffeinated drinks especially before going to sleep. You need to pay attention to the foods you eat before going to bedtime.

Many foods have certain substances in them that are natural and promote good quality of sleep.

Serotonin and Melatonin are two sleep-inducing hormones. These hormones also create a relaxing effect on our body.

What we can do is include the following foods in our diet to ensure that we get a good night's sleep.

The following foods will help you sleep better:

Snacks

Certain snacks like a banana with yogurt, apple, and mozzarella cheese, nuts like almonds and walnuts help in producing melatonin and serotonin. Eating these and even pistachios can all help in the production of serotonin and melatonin.

Fresh herbs

These can create a very calming effect on your body. Herbs like basil can make one feel tension free and help promote sleep. You can make basil and sage pasta sauce. Use this and feel the effect.

Do not consume black pepper or red pepper. They may cause a stimulating effect on your body.

Jasmine Rice

Choose to eat jasmine rice instead of eating normal rice. This rice can boost the levels of serotonin and tryptophan. A bowl of jasmine rice during dinner time should be able to give you a good night's sleep.

Milk

Warm milk or any dairy product for that matter which is low fat can help you fall asleep easily. Calcium helps induce sleep by helping to trigger melatonin. It also helps in regulating the movements of muscles.

Grapes

Fruits like grapes are capable of putting people to sleep after consumption. For people who suffer from insomnia, eating grapes can help them gain a good night's slumber. Eating grapes with yogurt can help release all stress, and one can easily fall asleep in the night.

Leafy greens

Eating spinach and Kale is a good solution to overcome slumber disorders. Including leafy greens in your diet is a healthy choice to gain sleep.

Dark chocolate

These have serotonin in them. Consuming them would help you induce sleep and keep your mind and body relaxed. For those who are health conscious, they should avoid eating dark chocolates that do not have milk in them.

Eggs

A great option to induce sleep. Eggs have a lot of nutrition in them which help induce sleep.

A Regular Sleep schedule for a happier, healthier life.

Erratic sleep patterns can leave you feeling out of whack, so a regular sleep schedule may be exactly what you need. Just a few adjustments to your daily routine can help you go to bed and wake up at the same time every day. These tips will help you take control of your internal clock.

Be Consistent.

Pick a bedtime and a wake-up time—and stick to them as much as possible. Life will inevitably interfere, but try not to sleep in for more than an hour or two, tops, on Saturdays and Sundays so that you can stay on track. That way, your body's internal clock—also called a [sleep_term id="1174"]—will get accustomed to a new bedtime, which will help you fall asleep better at night and wake up more easily each morning.

Make Gradual Adjustments.

You won't be able to change your sleep schedule overnight. The most effective tactic is to make small changes slowly. If you're trying to go to sleep at 10:00 pm, rather than midnight, for example, try this: For the first three or four nights, go to bed at 11:45 pm, and then go to bed at 11:30 pm for the next few days. Keep adjusting your sleep schedule like this. By working in 15-minute increments, your body will have an easier time adjusting.

See the Morning Light.

Your body's internal clock is sensitive to light and darkness, so getting a dose of the sun first thing in the morning will help you wake up. Opening the curtains to let natural light in your bedroom or having a cup of coffee on your sun-drenched porch will cue your brain to start the day.

Dim the Nightlights.

Likewise, too much light in the evenings can signal that you should stay awake. Before bedtime, dim as many lights as possible and turn off bright overhead lights. Avoid computers, tablets, cell phones, and TV an hour before bed, since your eyes are especially sensitive to the blue light from electronic screens. (If there's something good on TV at night, DVR it so you can watch it another time.)

Skip the Snooze Button.

Though it's certainly tempting to hit the snooze button in the morning to get a few extra winks, resist. The first few days of getting up earlier won't be easy, but post-snooze sleep isn't high quality. Instead, set your alarm to the time that you need to get up and remember that it may take a few minutes for your body to adjust to a daytime rhythm. If you can, skip the alarm altogether. Your body should wake up naturally after a full night's sleep—usually seven to nine hours—and you'll feel most alert if you wake up without electronic aid.

Food for Thought.

It's not just what you eat—it's when you eat. While you know that it's not a good idea to go to bed on an empty stomach, being stuffed is just as bad. Having dinner around the same time every night will help keep your whole body on track. Also, limit how much you drink before bedtime to avoid trips to the bathroom in the middle of the night. A good rule of thumb is to eat your last meal two to three hours before bedtime.

If you must eat before bed tries a small snack that blends carbohydrates and protein, such as cereal with a banana, cheese, and crackers, or wheat toast with natural peanut butter. You should also avoid nicotine, caffeine, and alcohol in the evenings since those stimulants take hours to wear off.

CHAPTER 4: BALANCED DIET FOR A HEALTHY AND BETTER LIFE

Maintaining a Balanced Diet

Keeping a healthy body is all about balance. Each of your body's systems constantly tries to stay in balance. It is this balance that keeps your body's systems functioning and your health stable.

Everyone has heard of the phrase "balanced diet." However, how many people know what that phrase means? What is a balanced diet?

There is no single path to a balanced diet. A balanced diet includes a daily mixture of foods from each of the basic food groups. The best way to guarantee that you are getting enough proteins, carbohydrates, fats, minerals, and vitamins is to eat different foods from each of the different food groups. Maintaining a balanced diet also means that balancing the food you eat with physical exercise. In other words, you have to eat the proper amount of calories for the amount of exercise you get. Doing this will help you maintain a healthy weight.

Keep in mind that the majority of people out there cannot

eat a perfectly balanced meal at every single meal. Keeping a truly balanced diet means balancing it for a week's worth of meals.

Who likes to eat the same food all the time? Nobody. If you choose a wide variety of healthy foods, it will help you maintain a balanced diet daily. So pick several different types of foods within each food group. Even if you love apples, try changing things up - eat a banana instead. Every week, make sure you are eating strawberries, cantaloupe, plums, nectarines, and grapes. Throw in mango or some kiwi every so often.

Fruits and vegetables play an important and vital role in a balanced diet. Nutritional powerhouses, they provide you with much-needed fiber, which also controls hunger. Vegetables are especially good for you. They are low in calories. They are also full of healthy phytochemicals which help stave off disease. Make sure you eat at least two helpings of vegetables and two helpings of fruit every day. Ideally, you should increase that number to three or four helpings. A helping should be half a cup or an entire fruit (excluding watermelons).

Balancing color is another tip for maintaining a balanced diet. Think of the colors of fruits and vegetables and make sure you are eating the entire spectrum. A simple way to ensure you are getting a solid mixture of vegetables and fruits is to eat as many colors in the rainbow as possible each week. Need red? Eat a strawberry. Want orange? Eat a... well, eat an orange. Yellow? Get some peaches and apricots. Need green? There are avocados, peas, broccoli, kiwi, and green beans. Blue? Blueberries. And purple? Eggplant, raisins, and elderberries. Every different color gives you a different nutrient, vitamin, mineral or antioxidant. So go ahead, eat the rainbow!

Bring these fruits and vegetables with you when you are on the go. Bring them to work or school or whenever you are in the car. This habit will keep your diet balanced and healthy and help cancel out any high-calorie, high-fat meals you may have at other times.

Don't like raw vegetables? Well, first of all, have you given them a chance? It may just be the thought of eating a raw vegetable that you don't like. They aren't as bland as you think they are. They are full of flavor. Try some now, especially if you haven't eaten any since you were a kid. You may find you like the taste and crunch now.

After trying them, if you still find you don't like the taste of raw vegetables, there is still hope. Try grilling them. This is a fast and simple way to make vegetables. Great vegetables to grill include peppers, zucchini, asparagus, onions, potatoes, eggplant, and mushrooms. Experiment with others to find your personal favorites. Grilled vegetables are great for side dishes or to put on top of pasta, rice, or pizza.

It is particularly important to eat a lot of vegetables and fruits while you are at home.

When you are at work or eating at a restaurant, you will have very few choices of vegetables and fruits. Sometimes you won't have any to choose from - especially if you find yourself at a fast food restaurant. If there are fruits and vegetables on the menu when you are eating out, then, by all means, order them. But often your only choice is to try to find something that has fewer calories and fewer amounts of sodium. If you manage to make these choices, you will have a better chance of maintaining a balanced flow of nutrients into your body.

Smoothies are an excellent way to get fruits and vegetables into your system without sacrificing taste.

If you fail to maintain a balanced diet, you will be at a greater risk for Type 2 diabetes, high blood pressure, and heart disease.

To achieve greater balance, exercise more and get more sleep. Add more physical activity to your daily routine. For example, if you are going out to lunch at work, walk there. And take the stairs. If you combine a balanced diet with healthy exercise, you will lose weight faster. Also, research proves that getting the proper amount of sleep will help you stay healthier. Not only does proper sleep help your digestive system, when you are rested you will make better choices about the foods you eat.

Remember, weight loss is all about balance. Eat right, exercise, and sleep well.

Balanced Dieting

Balanced dieting provides adequate nutrients and energy for good health and proper maintenance of body weight. An ideal balanced food contains minerals, vitamins, carbohydrates, fibers, fats and proteins in right proportions.

Unbalanced diet causes malnutrition and a host of other nutritional deficiency diseases. Adequate diet burns excessive fat from the body, promoting healthy weight loss. Well, a balanced diet also contains small quantities of other minerals, called micronutrients, which play specific roles in metabolic reactions.

Food choices and habits determine your long term health and immediate state of mind. Balanced weight loss programs improve your physical, mental and spiritual health.

Benefits of Balanced Dieting

Balanced dieting prevents arthritis, cancer, heart disease, and osteoporosis. It also maintains healthy levels of cholesterol in the body, besides reducing high blood pressure. It strengthens your immunity protecting you from old age-related ailments.

Well, balanced foods reduce obesity and overweight issues. They also promote healthy eating habits. Balanced foods work best when combined with yoga and moderate exercises.

Balanced dieting helps you to rebound from stressful activities better. They encourage you to lead a healthy lifestyle.

How to Optimize Weight Loss

Dieting flushes out excess fat and unwanted toxins from your body. While following a balanced food regimen, avoid alcohol, smoking, fat meats, and fast foods. Alcohol and smoking fill your body with excessive contaminants.

Drink plenty of water and freshly squeezed citrus fruit juices. They purify your bloodstream, filling it with stress-busting vitamins. Go for high fiber diets. They reduce constipation and cut the risk of colon cancer.

Balanced dieting is convenient and easy to follow. They are

fortified with nutrients, are easy to cook and taste excellent. Balanced dieting can be followed by kids and pregnant ladies alike. In three weeks, you observe a drastic change in your body shape. Don't be surprised if your husband thinks of tying the knot with you again!

Essential Foods for a Balanced Diet

We are all familiar with the notion of eating right. There is so much information about all sorts of healthy foods and their calorie values. There is enough being written about how vitamins are good for us and what are the rich sources of this nutrient. But rarely do we get to know the approximate quantity that is required by the human body on a daily basis. What makes a balanced diet? To make it a little simple let's get an overview of what should make your daily dietary intake.

The key nutrients that are required for smooth functioning of the diet are proteins, fat, fiber, minerals, iron, carbohydrates, vitamins, and calcium. A diet that includes all these essential nutrients, in the proper portion, is known as a balanced diet. Based on the average calorie requirement for a male weighing 60 kilograms it is 2700, and for a female weighing 55 kilograms, it is 2100.

Different age and lifestyles demand more intakes of certain nutrients to counter the deficiency and restore the balance.

The following is the list of essential foods and nutrients that are recommended in the general dietary intake for an average person -

Chapatti/Rice: Carbohydrate is the most important fuel for the human body. It is the refined carbohydrates like sugar, white bread, sodas and other processed foods that make you gain weight and make you prone to diabetes and heart diseases. A daily meal should consist of 4-5 portions of carbohydrates in a day.

Milk or Dairy Products: Dairy is essential for calcium, protein, phosphorous and magnesium. Some recent studies even suggest that dairy can help you cut belly fat. A minimum serving of 1-2 glasses of dairy is required every single day.

Vegetables: Vegetables are the most important part of a balanced diet. A minimum of 3-5 servings of vegetables is required daily to get minerals, fiber, iron, and most vitamins. The fiber in vegetables also helps regulate the use of sugars in the human body while helping to keep hunger and blood sugar in check. Eating vegetables is also linked to weight loss.

Fruits: One should eat at least two fruits a day to fulfill the requirement of vitamins in the human body. Fruits besides providing essential vitamins boost immunity to keep away from infections with its anti-oxidant properties to destroy free radical.

Pulses/Poultry and Other Meat: They are the main source of protein. If you believe in the myth that eating extra protein will add muscle mass, then you are wrong. The human body rather processes according to the requirement of the muscle and the extra protein gets saved as fat in the fat cells. 2-3 servings are more than sufficient for daily protein intake.

Water: Human body is 70-75% water and forms the bulk of blood and tissue fluid and is therefore essential for transporting nutrients, hormones and waste products around the body. Water is also essential to help digest the food and generate the energy required for body movements and other physical activities. Minimum of 10-12 glasses are important for the normal functioning of the body.

Fat: Extremely important for absorption of vitamins in the body. It also helps maintain the elasticity of the skin. A person requires at least 4-5 teaspoons of oil/butter every day. So for all those people who consider fat as their enemy should start to reconsider and add it to their diet. The real enemies are the Trans-fat and Saturated fat usually found in processed food. Fat can also help you improve memory and build muscle.

Healthy Diet Plan for a Healthy Life

A healthy diet plan means a well-balanced diet plan. Having a well-balanced diet plan is the key to a healthy diet. Keeping healthy is the best thing that you can do for yourself. Eating what you need and nothing extra will not only give your body the nutrition it needs but will also spare your body the trouble of digesting unwanted food.

A healthy diet plan will have you eating green vegetables, fruits, and other food items. You must remember that you have to do without all the junk food if you want to follow a healthy diet plan.

Good diet plan

A healthy diet plan doesn't mean eat x, y, z and only x, y, z. It means eating what works for you.

Eat green vegetables: It is important to eat green vegetables for your body to get vital minerals, vitamins, and enzymes to help your body function better. Vegetables a low in calories as well.

Fruits: Eating fruits can help take care of your sugar cravings for the day and will give you important vitamins and minerals.

Nuts: The oil that you get from almond nuts is very

important in the functioning of your body.

Fish: Fish fatty oil like Omega-3 is very important for your body.

Breakfast: A healthy breakfast that includes two eggs is important as the first meal of the day will give you the fuel you need to kick start your day.

Have smaller meals: Having smaller meals that will keep you going for three hours is important as you can avoid putting on extra weight by doing so.

Including this in your diet plan or replacing your current diet with the above-mentioned items will enable you to have a healthy diet plan. Remember it is what you eat and when you eat and how much you eat that will give you a healthy body. It is not easy to say eat 200gms of meat or drinks two glasses of milk a day as what works on you may not work on someone else.

Balance act

Balancing your daily intake of protein, fat, carbohydrates and calories is important as too much of everything is not good.

Having too much protein a day can cause bad effects on your liver so eating how much you require which is about 1 gram per pound of body weight a day is a health and any more than that will harm your liver. Also, remember to drink plenty of water.

Fat burns fat. Yes, this is true and did you know that your body needs a certain percentage of fat for its optimal functioning. Eating fat does not make you put on fat. So include some fat in your diet say about 15% of your daily intake of food must be fat.

Carbohydrates early in the day are good and late in the day is bad as you can put on fat if you have it later in the day and it is good earlier in the day.

Intake of calories must be limited as too much will make you put on fat.

So these are the tips for a healthy diet plan.

Exercise and Balanced Diet for a Healthy Life

A combination of a good exercise regime and a balanced diet will produce lasting results of a healthy life. Exercise not only keeps a person fit but makes one feel good about oneself. As the sayings go, "a healthy body has a healthy mind" and "you are what you eat." Exercising regularly stimulates the brain to produce endorphin, a chemical that helps a person feel more relaxed and peaceful. A balanced diet is essential to maintain a healthy weight. Exercise and nutrition go hand in hand.

Studies have shown that aerobics exercises can make your bones strong which in turn helps you age better. Eating low fat, low carb and high protein diet can help achieve goals faster. Exercising regularly prevents the risk of developing heart diseases, diabetes and certain types of cancers. To ensure that you are exercising hard enough without straining your heart, calculate heart rate by using the heart rate calculator. The optimum workout requires the heartbeat to go up to 75% of heart rate which will burn a lot of calories in a little amount of time.

Basic exercises to get you started:

There are three basic components to all exercise routines; Aerobics, Strength training and Flexibility or Stretching.

Aerobics exercise: Walking, jumping and swimming are the best forms of aerobic exercise. Jump rope brings the heart rate up much faster than walking. Hence, ten minutes of jump-rope is equivalent to twenty minutes of walking. Swimming is considered as the only workout that allows all the muscle groups to work together simultaneously to burn maximum calories.

Strength Training: Weights and Pilates are known as muscle toning and strengthening workouts. Weight training should be done at least three times a week. Pilates is getting quite popular nowadays especially in western countries. It teaches control of mind and body and helps strengthen core muscles.

Flexibility exercises: Yoga and stretching. Yoga is known for relaxation. It calms anxiety and brings about a holistic approach to life. Stretching is highly recommended after every workout. It is a good way to prevent injuries and soothe tired and sore muscles.

Benefits of exercising:

The benefits of exercise are innumerable, to name a few:

• Increased brain performance

• Feel more energetic

• Releases stress

• Keeps diseases at bay

• Makes the heart stronger

• Removes anxiety and depression

Importance of a Balanced Diet:

A balanced diet will provide you the energy your body needs to function properly. It is important to maintain healthy eating habits so that your immune system is strong enough to fight illnesses. Poor diet can hinder the growth and development of children. Kids with bad eating habits are more likely to continue it for the rest of their lives.

Easy tips to follow:

A healthy diet is a composition of fresh fruits and vegetables, lean proteins, dairy, and whole grains. Here are some simple do's and don'ts to get you started.

• Don't fill yourself up with empty calories, like cakes and cookies, etc.

• Try to make every calorie count by obtaining them from the four major food groups.

• Prefer fresh fruits over store-bought juices.

• Try to eat six small meals instead of three large ones.

• Always eat a healthy snack between breakfast and lunch, and between lunch and dinner.

• Finally, have a small snack just before bedtime. That way you won't end up consuming large portions at each meal.

When starting a healthy lifestyle, do some homework on how to calculate heart rate for an optimum workout, find out the caloric intake required for your age and try to maintain a food journal in the beginning. Just keep yourself disciplined through exercise, maintain a balanced diet, and you can enjoy a happy life for many years to come. Start bringing a change today by living the healthy way.

Healthy Balanced Diet Plans for All Age Groups

A balanced diet, as well as physical exercise, has a big part in reaching long wholesome life. The actual increasing understanding of the effects of meals on wellness has made all of us diet conscious as well as left all of us confused within the land associated with nutrition. You want to satisfy the palate as well as eat wholesome as well. This particular often limits our diet.

The major nutrition for the physique are proteins, carbohydrate, as well as fat. These types of providing the physique with power for various capabilities like defeating of coronary heart, activity associated with muscles as well as the brain. Additionally, the body requirements vitamins, as well as minerals about its optimal working.

To get a balanced diet as well as nutrition you should choose meals from all recommended food groups (cereals, impulses, poultry as well as meat, whole milk and dairy food, fruits as well as vegetables share the actual bais of importance associated with diet plan). Consuming a diverse diet increases the probabilities that all your nutrient requirements will be fulfilled; hence it is crucial to take the balanced diet.

Eating the balanced diet means consuming different types of meals from some food groups and also the right amount of every one of these meals to get all of the essential nutrients necessary for good health without consuming extra calories. Even though everyone selects foods through among the same groups, the balanced diet is very flexible, as well as means various things to different individuals, because the huge assortment of meals found within every group enables personal options in dinner planning.

Balanced Diet

A healthy diet strategy will serve great stability of every of the daily food groups listed. Various men and women need numerous amounts of meals. Additional factors, for example, age, physical proportions, exercise level, intercourse will also modify the quantity of what you eat. Below can be a guide to supply you with a common concept of how much via each team you need to function for a wholesome diet.

Vegetables

Vegetables additionally type solid grounds for a healthy diet, especially deep eco-friendly, abundant as well as dark yellow-colored vegetables. Kids through 2 to 6 many years require three servings every day; teen women, older kids, energetic women, and nearly all men must have four portions; and guy teens, as well as energetic males, should have Five servings

Milk, Yogurt and Cheese

Whole milk, yogurt in addition to cheese tend to be wholesome especially when they are low-fat or even fat-free. People from all age ranges should eat 2 to 3 portions each day out of this group. Although these foods tend to be wholesome, individuals who more often help make choices such as dairy or even regular parmesan cheese and natural yogurt risk growing their cholesterol.

Meat, Chicken, Fish, Dry Beans, Eggs and Nuts

Choices out of this team tend to be healthy once the meats, as well as chicken, tend to be lean as well as low fat. High-fat choices could enhance the risk of creating high cholesterol levels. Kids 2 to six many years must have two servings per day for an entire of Five ounces. Daily. Teen ladies, older children, energetic ladies and the majority of men ought to consume Two servings every day for a complete associated with Six oz.; lively men, as well as man teenagers, should eat Three servings daily for any complete of 7 oz.

Fruits

Such as veggies, fresh fruits are basic to a wholesome diet. Kids Two to 6 must have two portions per day related to fresh, freezing or even processed fruit; teenagers, teen women, energetic ladies, and most guys should have Three portions; as well as male teens and energetic males must have four servings.

Healthy Eating Advice - Creating a Balanced Diet for Good Nutrition

Healthy eating refers to eating suitable foods in an appropriate quantity. It's what fuels our bodies, and helps us live longer lives, and fight off curable diseases.

Healthy Eating and Nutrition

Healthy eating is vital to living a harmonious and balanced life. It prevents damage to your body's cells and even keeps your skin soft and smooth.

If you consume a high level of sweets, it will lower your immune system defenses. Therefore, it is essential to consume those kinds of foods in moderation, or better yet, just eliminate them from your diet.

On the opposite end of the food spectrum, proper nutrition must be followed. Eating a balanced diet gives enough nourishment to stay fit, as long as you combine it with regular exercise.

When you practice healthy eating and nutrition, it will end the majority of your health problems, allowing you to live healthier. In this age of rapid rising health care costs, staying healthy can have a positive effect on your family's finances. A poor diet of fatty, processed foods leads to obesity, which can rapidly turn into health problems, and extra medical expenses.

Healthy eating is a lifelong commitment that requires discipline and changing your eating patterns. Try consuming plenty of leafy green vegetables that contain high levels of vitamins and minerals.

Consuming fast food, sweets, and processed food does not contribute to healthy eating patterns, and it will erode your body's nutritional level, allowing it to fall to disease.

An Apple a Day

Consuming enough fruits will ease the everyday load on your digestive system. Fruits are highly rich in vitamins and fiber. Fruit provides enough natural sugars to eliminate your cravings for other sweets. You can keep your system clean and healthy by consuming a lot of fruit each day.

Become a Healthy Vegetarian

Some people think that becoming a vegetarian is an extreme form of nutrition. Also, there are many people who still don't believe it's possible to obtain enough protein and healthy fats from being a vegetarian.

To set the record straight, if you load up on rice, nuts, and grains, you will have more than enough protein. The fact is, most Americans, and folks of other nationalities eat too much protein. You can easily eat too much protein, but it's very difficult to eat enough fruits and vegetables.

Eat in Moderation

Never eat a lot of food at one sitting. It's better to eat 4-6 smaller portions throughout the day. A hearty breakfast can keep you going through the day, and should never be skipped. However, your dinner should be eaten early to avoid putting an extra strain on your digestive system while you are trying to sleep.

Exercise and More Exercise

Exercise is probably the best way of keeping a person fit and healthy. Getting enough exercise goes hand-in-hand with healthy eating, and the combinations of the two are the best way to keep you fit and healthy. Proper exercise also helps regulate your eating habits. You are not as hungry after a good workout, and the calories you burn while exercising helps you lose weight faster.

CHAPTER 5: REGULAR EXERCISE HELPS ACHIEVE BETTER LIVING

Fitness and Your Health

Being physically active is a vital part of being healthy for any individual. Eating a balanced, healthy diet and being active in your daily life are the two best things to help you keep healthy and young. Everyone should try to get in at least three days a week where they are doing some sort of exercise, although more is better.

Weight-bearing exercise is important for some individuals, especially those who are suffering from bone loss, or have a history of bone loss in their family. Doing weight lifting exercises puts pressure on your bones which helps them to grow stronger. Other people who might want to do weight lifting exercises are those who want to have well-defined muscles or people who have sagging skin. Lifting weights will improve the overall look of your body by toning and tightening it up. Using light weights can still be effective for this, as long as you feel some burn while you are working out.

If you desire to use heavier weights, there is no need for

women to be afraid of becoming manly looking? It takes a long time and a lot of weights to get the look that most female bodybuilders possess. Studies have shown that weight-bearing exercise is just as beneficial to the heart as cardiovascular exercise. Weight lifting exercises should be done at least three times per week, and each body part should never be trained back to back.

Cardio exercise helps you lose weight, lower your chance of heart attack, lower blood pressure, and improve your mood and lower stress levels. Cardio exercise should be done about five times per week for maximum results. You should choose the type of exercise that you enjoy.

Good ideas for cardio exercises include biking, walking, jogging, playing tennis, playing basketball, skating, and inline skating, swimming, and skiing and team sports. You can also use cardio as a type of functional exercise. This means instead of driving to the grocery store, try walking instead. This way you aren't going out of your way to fit in exercise, but you are still reaping the benefits. You should try to do cardio for at least half an hour, and try to make sure you raise your heart rate a little.

Before engaging in any type of exercise, you should get a complete physical examination to make sure you aren't suffering from heart disease or some other type of illness. After your doctor gives you the green signal to start exercising, start slow and work your way up. Remember always; exercise should be fun and enjoyable. If you chose something you find boring, chances are you won't stick with it.

Exercise to Boost Your Health and Improve Your Fitness

The late fitness expert Jack LaLanne once said that "exercise is king, nutrition is queen, put them together and you've got a kingdom." But if you are leading a sedentary lifestyle and just eat what you want regardless if the food is nutritious or not, then you are not building your fitness kingdom.

For the longest time, people in the United States and elsewhere around the world have been eating unhealthy fast food and processed food but have been very little or even zero exercise to get rid of the excess calories that they consume. This unhealthy lifestyle has led to increasing global obesity rates.

Here is proof that a sedentary lifestyle (which is just a euphemism for sitting down all day doing nothing) will make you fat and unhealthy: a study published in Clinical Cardiology revealed that morbidly obese people walked less than 2,500 steps a day and remained sedentary for more than 99 percent of the time (walking 10,000 steps daily is recommended for a healthy lifestyle).

There is no doubt about it: exercise and the proper diet are pillars of good health and fitness. Sadly, more than half of all adults in America do not get the recommended amount of exercise. Alarmingly, 25 percent do not get any exercise at all. Nutrition, the queen of the fitness kingdom, is also being ignored. If you watched the documentary Super Size Me, you would realize that you must be smarter about your food choices if you want to stay fit and healthy.

The Benefits of Exercise and Good Nutrition

Stop saying that you do not have time to work out and shop for nutritious food. You should start thinking that exercise is every bit as important as breathing, good nutrition, and sleeping. Working out should not be seen as a leisure activity or a luxury; it should be viewed as part of your regular schedule.

Here are some of the most profound benefits of exercise to your physical fitness:

Trimming Your Belly Fat

Regular moderate to high-intensity aerobic workouts have the biggest impact on reducing belly fat, also known as abdominal fat and visceral fat, the dangerous type of fat that increases your risk of cardiovascular disease, certain types of cancer, and type 2 diabetes.

Controlling Calories

You need to use up more calories than you consume if you want to lose weight. Working out regularly helps you burn extra calories that would otherwise be deposited in your body as fat.

Keeping Extra Pounds Off

About 90 percent of people who have experienced weight loss and were able to keep it off for a year do about an hour of physical activity a day.

Boosting Your Metabolism

You can lose weight if you go on a diet without working out, but you will also lose muscle mass, which means that you will burn a lesser amount of calories. Doing strength training allows you to build muscle mass and boost your metabolism, which allows you to burn more calories.

Curbing Your Hunger

If you go on a diet and work out at the same, you will find that you are less hungry than if you only diet.

Effective Exercises for Fitness

It is important to execute fitness exercise as one of your priorities since it is the key to good health and a better lifestyle. Exercising is an essential part of any fitness program, but not all exercises are the same, and some are just more effective than others.

Efficient exercises not only cover more muscle groups, but they also take less time to do than wrong exercises that do not serve the purpose. When it comes to fitness, there are five exercises that are especially effective and which can easily be done.

1. Walking. If you are looking for an exercise that does a lot, then it is walking. It works on various muscles, especially in the legs, and it also does wonders for your cardiovascular system. The speed, distance and amount of time spent walking should be suitable for your fitness level, and

whenever you can complete a tour with ease, you can step things up a notch and once again improve your fitness. With walking as an option, there is no reason fitness cannot be part of your daily program. All you need for a walk is a good pair of shoes.

2. Crunches. This is an effective exercise that can be done anyplace and which helps improve your fitness. They are necessary because they target muscles that are otherwise not targeted by other forms of exercise, no matter how good and effective they are for other things. Crunches are also an essential part of strength training which you will have to work on to be fit.

3. Squats. A big part of any fitness program is strength training and squats are perfect for the job. When you do squats, you will be using a lot of muscle groups at the same time. Once again you can do squats anywhere, so there is no excuse not to include this effective exercise in your program.

4. Interval training. This is the best way to improve overall fitness. It involves mixing various effective exercises and then alternative the speed in which you perform them.

5. Jump rope. The jump rope is probably one of the best tools you can find to help you with your fitness training. It is an effective exercise because it targets muscles and strengthens your heart. If you can keep up with this exercise

for a few minutes at a fast pace, then you know that you have a good fitness level.

Few Tips for better Exercise

Exercising for fitness and weight loss is a formula for health that cannot be denied. But how does one get started on this path which ultimately leads to good health? The American College of Sports Medicine recommends 30 minutes of moderate intensity physical activity at least five days per week. Or vigorous intensity activity at least three days per week. Add in strength training at least two times during a week. Here are Five tips on how you can begin to incorporate physical activity into your daily regimen.

1) Schedule it. Give yourself a set time frame for when you'll do your exercise. This should be the same time each day that you work out so that it becomes part of your daily routine.

2) Do it in short spurts. The physical activity can be cumulative. The activity of moderate intensity can be amassed throughout the day, preferably in 10-minute intervals, which lead to a total of 30 minutes.

3) Alter the approach. You can alternate between moderate and vigorous intensity activity during the week. As an example, you could ride a stationary bike at vigorous intensity three times a week, and walk briskly at moderate intensity the other two days of the week.

4) The family that plays together stays together. Bring along your wife and the kids on your exercise routine. This can add enjoyment to the routine as well as prepare the children for a lifetime of being fit.

5) Use your imagination. There are a variety of activities you can use to keep from becoming bored with any physical activity. Such as tennis, paddle ball, swimming, and bowling just to name a few.

Combine this with a reduction in daily caloric intake, and you've got a formula for fitness and weight loss guaranteed for success

7 Uncommon Tips for Exercising

Studies have shown that regular exercise is a significant factor in living a long and healthy life. According to a study performed at Harvard University, people that exercise daily have several benefits opposed to those that do not. Some of these benefits are improved sleep, prevents weight gain and reduces the risk of falling among older adults. Although to some this may seem like common knowledge, sometimes it may be difficult to know where to start and how to continue exercising every day. The following tips will help you as you begin and continue exercising daily.

1. Commit to your exercise plan

Starting any activity or goal is easy; finishing that activity or goal is the difficult part. Before you begin exercising make sure that your exercise goals are realistic. Choose activities that are enjoyable to you and schedule out a week of activities. In this schedule indicate which activities you will perform on which days and stick to it.

The more that you exercise and build muscle the easier exercising will become. However, starting and stopping every few months or even weeks doesn't provide the sustained growth that exercising every day does. So when you make your exercise goals and plans make sure that it is a plan that you can commit to.

2. Start Slow and Gradually Increase your Level of Activity

When beginning exercising decide where you are at with your physical fitness and begin slowly and increase your activity as your level of fitness increases. Avoid generalized workouts because they are designed to work for as many people as possible. What works for someone else might not work for someone you.

Don't get stuck in a rut continue to progress and make the exercises challenging. As your body grows in strength and endurance activities that were once challenging will no longer be as challenging. An important part of exercising is challenging your body to achieve more each time. This is how sustained muscle growth is achieved.

3. Save Stretching For Last

Think of your body like a rubber band that has been placed in a freezer. When you take that rubber band out of the freezer and try to stretch it, the rubber band breaks. The same thing applies to our muscles and bodies. They take time to warm up; that is why it is important to stretch throughout your exercising.

Many people believe that they should stretch before they perform an activity. However recent studies have proven this to be incorrect. "It has been a long time since anyone has recommended extensive stretching before exercise because it has been known for a while now that the best time to stretch is after," said Richard Cotton, the national director of certification at the American College of Sports Medicine.

If you decide to go on a walk or run wait to stretch your muscles until after you have finished. This time gives your muscles a chance to loosen up a little bit and will make your stretching more beneficial for your overall mobility. Stretching can be a great tool to help with overall mobility but only when done right and at the right time.

4. Don't Exercise With a Friend...

Having someone interested in your exercise goals can help you to be motivated to accomplish those goals. Even if you don't have a desire to exercise with someone you should explain your exercise goals to family members and friends so they can help you with the process. Having someone to help motivate and encourage is a good way of having exercise success.

Another aspect of exercising with a friend is the social aspect of exercising. Sometimes it's just good to have someone to talk to when you wake up for that early morning walk, jog or weight training session.

5. Don't Exercise Painfully

The old saying of 'no pain, no gain' should not be considered when exercising. Reasons vary for why people want to exercise, but for the most part, it is to become healthy. Stop anytime during exercise when you feel pain. The last thing that you want to do is to hurt yourself and not be able to perform daily tasks or to continue exercising daily.

6. Hydrate

One of the best ways to overcome illness or recover from an injury is to hydrate; the same thing applies when exercising. When you exercise you lose water through perspiration that water needs to be replenished.

According to Webmd.com, you should be drinking six or eight 8-ounce glasses of water every day (48-64 ounces) and 8 ounces for every 15 minutes exercise.

To help you stay hydrated check out the Hydra-Paks found at Stander.com

7. Don't get discouraged

Anytime that people start a new routine in their lives they will be faced with days where they don't want to continue the routine. This especially applies when beginning a new exercise routine. The important thing to remember is to continue to push through the times of discouragement. Having help from family members and friends to help motivate you is a good way of overcoming this discouragement.

Weekly Plan Overview – Exercise to Reduce Whole- Body Inflammation

FIRST WEEK

SATURDAY: 30 min. Light Exercise

SUNDAY: Light Circuit

MONDAY: 30 min. Moderate Exercise

TUESDAY: REST

WEDNESDAY: 30 min. Moderate Exercise

THURSDAY: Light Circuit

FRIDAY: REST

SECOND WEEK

SATURDAY: 30 min. Light Exercise

SUNDAY: Light Circuit

MONDAY: 30 min. Moderate Exercise

TUESDAY: REST

WEDNESDAY: 30 min. Moderate Exercise

THURSDAY: Light Circuit

FRIDAY: REST

THIRD WEEK

SATURDAY: 30 min. Light Exercise *Yoga*

SUNDAY: Light Circuit *weights all over*

MONDAY: 30 min. Moderate Exercise *Cardio Sweat or at work either is good*

TUESDAY: REST

WEDNESDAY: 30 min. Moderate Exercise *off work*

THURSDAY: Light Circuit *off work*

FRIDAY: REST

FOURTH WEEK

SATURDAY: 30 min. Light Exercise

SUNDAY: Light Circuit

MONDAY: 30 min. Moderate Exercise

TUESDAY: REST

WEDNESDAY: 30 min. Moderate Exercise

THURSDAY: Light Circuit

FRIDAY: REST

CHAPTER 6: A BETTER LIFE WITH HEALTHY RELATIONSHIPS

Are You in Healthy Relationships?

As hard it is to believe, there are few people who are in healthy relationships, and there are some who are in an unhealthy relationship, and they do not know or even realize it. They have come from one unhealthy relationship to the next until they can hardly recognize an unhealthy relationship even if it hit them in the face. Healthy relationships are vital for the health of both the people in the relationship both mentally, psychological and physical. Healthy relationships are where the partners love each other unconditionally. When they are together what they do is have fun. Yes, they do argue, but the number of times they argue with each other is far much less than the number of times they are in good terms with each other.

People in healthy relationships respect each other. Whatever the partner decides to do on their own is respected by the other partner. Even if the decision made by the other person is not entirely agreeable to them, they will still respect each other's opinion and come to an agreement or a compromise. They will also respect each other when their friends and family are around and will never do anything to make the other person feel ashamed before someone else. There also exists a lot of honesty in a healthy relationship. The partners know everything about each other but still, love each other. If anyone did something wrong, they would also be honest enough to admit they did it.

Trust also exists in healthy relationships. You cannot say to be in a healthy relationship if you cannot trust a person. You can go out all by yourself and leave your partner behind, and they will trust you enough to know that you cannot do anything to hurt them. There should also be some level of good communication between you and your partner. If your partner is the type to keep quiet about things that directly affect your relationship, then you are not in a healthy relationship. The two of you should be able to talk about the things that affect the two of you in any way. Embarrassing or otherwise.

A healthy relationship is one where the two of you can be yourselves and have nothing to hide about. A healthy relationship is one where there is general support. It is not about every man or woman for himself and God for all of you. In healthy relationships, couples support each other in all ways. Be it financially, physically, emotionally and any kind of support that is needed. No one in the relationship is afraid to ask for help just because they think they will look weak and the partner might end up looking down upon them. Everyone needs help once in a while, even the strongest ones of them sometimes need to get help. A healthy relationship is one where a partner is not afraid to ask for it and will not feel guilty about asking for it neither will they feel like they are disturbing their partner. That is as long as it is something you need help in.

Interacting with People

Interacting with other people is a way to socialize or create a network. Either you talk to a person or write; wave to someone; approach or go near and look at a man or a woman, it is a way of interacting. The difficulty of it depends on the purpose.

There are different reasons why people socialize. Some reasons are very simple while others are complicated. One simple reason is when you need to ask for direction. A complicated case is when applying for a job. But whether simple or complicated the purpose of a man for interacting is, it is no doubt necessary. And that I think is the hardest thing - having to interact because of necessity.

A person needs to communicate and mingle with other people to live. You have to speak to a vendor to trade for food. A person has to exchange ideas with others to grow and become successful in life. You must listen and learn from mentors or teachers to achieve your dreams. One has to rely on somebody else to survive. You should see and consult a doctor when ill. To be able to reach its destination, one has to talk to someone even if the person is a total stranger. You need to call a driver to go to a place. Therefore, whether they like it or not, every human will interact all of the time.

So, even if the person you need to talk to is a difficult person to deal with, you need to face the consequence, either good or bad. What if you do not have the skills to handle this kind? It is going to be unmanageable. And what if you do not speak the same language? You certainly will not understand one another. What if you do not share the same culture? You might misinterpret each other. What if you are not so fluent in communication? You may be misunderstood. And so many "what if" that you need to face and resolve just to be able to interact well and serves its purpose.

Hence no matter why and how you are interacting, the mere fact that it is necessary is what makes it difficult. Because it is a necessity, you must do what is required to be able to communicate well. It is hard to study, but it is required to easily cope with the fast-changing world. To improve your communication skills is quite difficult, but it is essential to have a good interpersonal relationship. To develop your personality and become a better person for socialization and career growth is an elaborated task, but truly rewarding. To go on training so you can hone your skills and build up self-confidence, to establish a larger network that will contribute to your success can be tiring but is worth doing.

Be it a person you know - a friend, relative, classmate, cyber pal, your teacher, a colleague at work, boss, customer, business partner, prospective client, etc., or a stranger; they can be important people you will have to deal with. And if you are ready because you are well equipped with the requirements needed to fit in, the acts or move you take with them will not be at all that hard.

How to Connect with People

It is so rewarding to know how to connect with people. It is true that people are the most important asset. Poet and author Ralph Waldo Emerson, asserted, "Assets make things possible, people make things happen."

Connecting with people can make the difference in your leadership, in your family, in your business, in your vision, in your department or organization. Don't ever underestimate the power of connecting with people. The former American president, Theodore Roosevelt saw the value of connecting with people, and he remarked, "The most important single ingredient in the formula of success is knowing how to get along with people."

Let me share with you ways that you can follow to connect with people.

Respect people

The fundamental requirement to connect with people is that you must respect them. Solid relationships start with respect. If there is no respect, then there is no relationship or connection. You can go anywhere in the world, and you will find that no one connects to someone who does not respect him or her.

Respect is about valuing people as they are, not by their abilities. You respect the fact that they are normal human beings. When people feel valued and respected by you, they will have confidence in you, and they will easily connect with you.

Respect for people is not determined by someone's background, race, ethnicity, sexuality, education, achievements, affiliation, religion, culture, and nationality. But it is determined by the worth of having been made in the image of God. Respect people for who they are and they will appreciate it and get connected to you.

Show people that you genuinely care

Show people that you genuinely care by greeting, interacting and asking them how they are doing. Ask them how their family, kids, parents or spouse are doing. When they happen to be in an emotionally charged situation like the death of the loved one or any kind of lose, offer your sincere support.

People connect easily with those who genuinely show that they care. The founder of the red cross, the late Mother Theresa said, "Being unwanted, unloved, uncared for, forgotten by everybody, I think that is a much greater hunger, much greater poverty than the person who has nothing to eat."

Make people feel important

People want to feel recognized and important. The key to making people feel important is to appreciate them both privately and publicly whenever they do something good. Appreciation makes people feel like they are contributing something of value to the family, ministry, community, team, division, department, business or organization. It makes them feel important.

People will connect with those who sincerely appreciate their diligent contribution to the good course. If you want to connect with people, make them feel important and special.

Look for potential in people

Every person has potential. If you want to connect with people, look for potential in people. Successful people look at others to see the best that is in them. When you show people that you have identified the potential in them, they will see that you believe in their best. And they will connect with you.

When you look at people with the eye of finding potential in them, you put yourself in a situation to make a difference in their lives. Connect with people by looking for potential in them and by motivating and showing them how to bring it out.

Smile

A smile is the most brightening thing that brightens the atmosphere. Smile beautifies life. It is very attractive. It is inviting, and it brings life and happiness. When somebody genuinely smiles at you, you get connected to him or her. A smile is a powerful force that enables one to connect with people. It makes one's face shine with warmness.

Smiling at people when you communicate with them, gets them connected to you and your message. People enjoy being around people who express faith and hope in life through their smile. If you want to connect with people, lighten up your face with a sincere smile.

Learn people's names

A name to a person is his or her most important and sweetest sound. Learning people's names is the most important thing you can ever do. When you call somebody by name, he or she will feel sweet and important inside, and they will get connected to you.

Adjust the tone of your voice

The tone of your voice determines the atmosphere of your communication with people. J. A. Holmes said, "Ninety percent of the friction of daily life is caused by the wrong tone of voice."If your tone is not warm, it will be hard for people to get connected to you. When your tone is warm when you communicate a particular message to people, they will act warmly toward you.

It is very important to learn how to adjust the tone of your voice in any given situation so that you don't push people away when you must draw them closer to you. Don't ever project a wrong tone in your interactions with people. Let the tone of your voice be right at all times.

Be a good listener

Listening is a powerful skill that enables people to connect with others. Leadership guru and author John C Maxwell said, " The ability to skillfully listen is the foundation to building positive relationships with others." Great people understand that being a good listener is the most valuable thing that leads to success in relationships.

When you listen to people with an intent to understand their message, frustrations, pain, hurt or their concern, you will get connected to them. Listening shows care and respect. Be a good listener, and you will connect with people.

Embrace empathy

Empathy is the ability to put yourself in people's shoes. It is the ability to one's imagination to feel people's pain, to experience what they are experiencing to understand what they are going through. Humanity theorist Carl Rogers said, "If you want to understand people, get into their phenomenal world, experience what they are experiencing, and you will know how to communicate help to them."

Empathy enables people to understand the pain, frustrations and the hurt that others are going through to the extent that they do something to help. When you are empathic, people will get connected to you because they will feel that you care and you see them as important. They will have confidence in you.

Be humble

Humble people always have a way of connecting with people. Humility is about the ability to subordinate yourself to proper principles, values, and morals. When you are humble, you are not full of yourself. Humble people put the interests and needs of other people ahead of their interests and needs.

Benjamin Franklin said, "If you want to lose friends quickly, start bragging about yourself; if you want to make and keep friends, start bragging about others." People get connected to those who are humble. If you want to be connected to people, humble yourself. Don't allow pride to stand on your way of establishing strong relationships with people.

Connecting with people is the foundation for success in building great relationships. People are of higher value and importance. They have the potential to add value to you if you can learn how to connect with them.

Healthy Relationships - How to Develop Them

There are many people whose preference is to have healthy, happy relationships with the people in their lives... whether they are parent-child relationships, marriage or love relationships, family relationships, friendships, or even relationships with work colleagues. Building healthy relationships is a normal and natural desire. Healthy relationships are a vital aspect of mental health, and general health and wellness. So what do we need to know about building and maintaining healthy relationships?

Let us define some of the qualities of healthy relationships:

• Each person takes responsibility for their own needs

• You can easily discuss conflict and differences, without blame

• The relationship is important to each person involved

• Each person communicates openly and honestly

• Abuse is absent -- this includes physical, verbal, or emotional abuse

• Each person has healthy boundaries -- can say "no" to requests without feelings of guilt

Certainly, it is important for each party in a relationship to understand, and be able to practice these aspects when interacting with others. It is my belief, however, that the key to healthy relationships is found, first, in our interactions with our Self, with our Inner Being.

What is your relationship like with your Inner Being?

- Are you in conflict with yourself?

- Do you ever heap blame on yourself?

- Do you get angry or frustrated with yourself?

- Is your relationship with your Inner Being important to you?

- Do you communicate openly and honestly with your Inner Being?

- Do you abuse yourself...with thoughts or words?

- Can you follow your inner guidance without feeling guilty?

If your relationship with your Inner Being is not a healthy one, then keeping up a healthy relationship with others in your life could be challenging for you. The relationship you have with your Inner Being is the most important relationship you will ever have... and every other relationship is a reflection (in some way) of that most intimate, inner one.

Do you ever feel angry or frustrated with yourself, or blame and criticize yourself? Your Inner Being never argues with you, or blames you, or gets angry or frustrated or disappointed with you... your Inner Being always beams pure, positive, love energy to you -- without exception. If you blame or criticize yourself, then you conflict with your Inner Being -- and you feel that tension through negative emotions.

Do you value your relationship with your Inner Being? Is it important for you to feel good, and feel happy? When you value your relationship with your Inner Being, then you make every effort you can to feel happy and to focus your attention on thoughts that feel good when you think them.

Do you communicate honestly and openly with your Inner Being? This is as easy as tuning in to your emotions. Your emotions give you feedback about your relationship with your Inner Being...when you feel positive, happy emotions, then you are in tune with your Inner Being. Negative emotions show that you are thinking of something that does not agree with what your Inner Being knows.

Do you take time to nurture your relationship with your Inner Being? Do you nurture and soothe yourself? There are many ways you can nurture your spirit...you can meditate or listen to soothing music. You can also nurture yourself by thinking of someone you love or taking a warm bath, or by taking a walk, or by just giving yourself permission to chill...just for a moment.

Do you abuse yourself with thoughts or words? It always feels good to receive support and encouragement from others...but we can also be supportive and encouraging toward ourselves. This can mean not asking or demanding too much of ourselves in time and effort -- by realizing that you don't have to do whatever-it-is this minute. We can applaud our efforts, and focus on what we did right (and not what went wrong).

Can you follow your Inner Guidance without feeling guilty? Do you trust your emotions and your 'gut' feelings? I have noticed that when I follow my 'gut' feelings and trust my emotions, my path always leads to new and improved experiences -- I feel inspired, and creative, and passionate, and alive.

So...what is your relationship like with your Inner Being?

If you make an effort to improve your relationship with your Inner Being and make it a healthy one, then every other relationship in your experience will also improve, and you will enjoy healthy relationships.

Top Ten Rules for a Happy Relationship

We all want that fairy tale story when we enter a new relationship. In the beginning, it's all laughs and giggles. We wake up every morning anticipating another day to see he or she's faced, or hear their voice. No one gets into a relationship and thinks "A year from now it will change?" The fact of the matter is it does change; it's up to you to save it. It's not all raindrops and gumdrops. Most relationships fail because people are so quick to give up on each other over the littlest things when they're not as happy as much as they were in the beginning. Relationships aren't easy, and I'm not going to pretend that is! When it boils down to it, we all want happiness.

There are a lot of things you can do to save your relationship and keep it on the fast track so let's begin. I'm going to tell you ten things to keep a happy relationship, some of these tips may be obvious, but if you were using them to your advantage you wouldn't be reading this article right? So here we go ten rules to having a happy relationship:

1. Patience - Learn to always be positive in your relationship and practice patience. By patience I mean learn to comprise with your partner even when you feel that you have none

left. Be patient

2. Communication - One major problem in relationships is communication. Communication is one of the key things to keep a relationship strong and to go. Always express how you feel good or bad. Tell your partner and then discuss the issue and resolve it. You will be amazed at how much you can learn from each other by communicating.

3. Trust - Let me just say this without trust a relationship will fail. If you are in a relationship, you must have this. Don't assume anything, always communicate as I stated in step 2. Insecurity and jealousy are not safe in a relationship. Being a mother or a father to your partner won't work. If you have any doubts ask, but don't assume. Trust your partner; if your partner values your trust, then you shouldn't be worried about anything trust me.

4. Friends - Be friends with your partner. Learn about the stuff he or she likes and take a liking to it. So even if you're not interested to act like it. Be their buddy first; a relationship is not a job, let loose and have fun together you'd be surprised.

5. Spontaneous - Do random, unexpected things together. Surprise your partner with a night out or with random gifts or text or calls. Being spontaneous shows that you want to add excitement to your relationship and that he or she is

worth trying new things with and for.

6. Space - No one likes someone who is always in their space. Give your partner space; you don't always have to be together every day. Give yourself enough space to miss each other. Go out with friends from time to time. You don't always have to be with your partner 24/7 it gets boring, and that's how arguments occur. Learn to miss each other.

7. Don't Criticize - Never past judgment on your partner. You are their biggest supporter; learn to be there for them even if you disagree. Agree to disagree for them.

8. Public Display of Affection - Showing that you love your partner in public means a lot to them. Grabbing his or her hand, putting your arm around them or even kissing them shows them that you love them and don't care who sees and knows

9. Sex - You thought I wasn't going to mention this? Yes, sex plays a major part in a relationship. So don't be boring! Learn what your partner likes and doesn't like and do it. Role play, dirty talk, even watching porn together it's erotic. To me the more spontaneous it is, the better. Sex and relationships go hand in hand.

10. Privacy- Learn to keep your relationship problems to yourself. Never let outsiders no your business and put things in your head. People always have an opinion good or bad.

Only you know what you and your partner have so no outsider can tell you otherwise. Don't put your problems on social networks many relationships fail due to social networks. Keep your private life off the internet.

Relationships aren't perfect, but love is a beautiful thing to share it.

CHAPTER 7: STAY HAPPY FOR A GOOD LIFE

Happiness Is a Choice

Happiness is a skill and the habits I will be sharing will energize you to acquire a high happiness level. Do you find yourself wondering what would make you truly happy? We live in a world where we are taught that making money, becoming successful or becoming famous makes one happy. Social media tells you that someone else around you is happier than you. So maybe you work very hard, waiting for your vacation, for a slice of that happiness. I want you to know that you have everything it takes to be happy in your present condition. Happiness does not lie in the pursuit or a future moment. Happiness, like your time in those days, includes completely engaging in an activity with others and the moment. Have you ever had the opportunity of watching a baby find happiness? I watch my nephew laugh at a song, at a funny face, at a shift in an ordinary moment. We have this ability to laugh when we allow ourselves to experience the awe and pleasure of a newborn. Why should you be happy? I linked happiness to long life, increase in energy, success and even more positive marriages. When we practice happiness, they are linked to positive health outcomes. Studies show that happy people are more likely to experience better marriages, promotions at work and life satisfaction. Happy states have been shown to contribute to mental flexibility and creativity.

You may be asking if some people are born happier than others. Research shows that happiness is a function of your genetic predisposition, circumstances that you face, and the choices that you make. The interplay of these factors will result in a gain or lack of happiness. The good news is, if you had "unhappy" genes, you could make up for them by choosing habits that result in happiness. Some circumstances in your life may or may not be changed. Heavier weighted happiness factors are products of genetics and choices. You can't change the genes you were given, so let's discuss the choices you make which have been shown to produce happy moments.

You can choose to live a happy lifestyle. Every day, even when you do not feel like it, you can commit to be happy. Then practice and keep practicing. I don't want you to chase happiness. I want you to choose habits each day that will lead you to feel happy. What should happiness look like? It is not giggling or grinning senselessly every day. Happiness can include states of contentment, calmness, the ability to sit with difficult moments and the feeling that you are in charge of your environment. You can practice happy habits each day, and like any goal, you can start with a commitment to lead a happy life. Happiness is not something I want you to strive for. Happiness is found in the daily moments and not in striving or wishing "I want to be happy." Martin Seligman, a leader in the field of Positive Psychology and Happiness, explained that you could find happiness by choosing a combination of positive emotions, engaging in things you value, finding meaning in your life, engaging in relationships and accomplishments. These skills can be practiced to cultivate states of happiness. We can take action each day to contribute to this area in our lives.

How to Find Happiness That Comes From Within

Life isn't always a bed of roses. And regardless of your circumstances, there will be times when it appears that things just aren't going the way you want them to. Even though you may be down in the dumps, or having your own 'pity party,' there are countless people living fascinating and extraordinary lives.

This may cause you to ask the question, "how do they manage to live such extraordinary lives? Are they even bothered by the stress of a busy life?" But the fact is, they know a secret that most people have, but don't use. They know they must work on themselves and discover how to find happiness from within.

So the million dollar question is, "how do you find happiness?" What does it take to be genuinely happy? The first step is to love yourself. I once heard that "loving means accepting." When you start to truly love yourself, it means that you accept your imperfections. No one is perfect. You need to be courageous to discover ways to accept your mistakes and learn from them.

Next, there's being content. To be genuinely happy, you have to be content. Some people mistake contentment as complacency. This is not so. When you're content with the way you earn an income, your looks, your family, your friends, where you live, your vehicle, and all the various things in your life - right now, without waiting for 'someday,' this is the beginning of genuine happiness.

Think of life as one big lab experiment. It's all about finding out what's right and what's wrong — trying and failing and winning and losing. All types of events will occur as often as you inhale and exhale. Failure, in your life, may be plentiful, but don't let this prevent you from being happy.

Then there's the mistaken belief that materials things are an express road to happiness. This is the furthest thing from being true. Happiness has never been about acquiring material things, owning dream vehicles or becoming an employee of the year.

The game of life is never fair. Sometimes, life's most sought after prizes don't always go to the fastest, the strongest, the bravest or not even the best. One surefire way to find happiness is to create your definition of what happiness means to you.

Happiness for an author could be selling a million copies of their book. Happiness for a basketball rookie may mean getting the rookie of the year award. Happiness for a homeless person may mean living in a one bedroom apartment. It's different for everyone. So don't feel as though you need to have the best of everything to be happy.

Authentic happiness is about doing and making the best out of small things. When you catch yourself smiling at your mistakes and saying to yourself "Oh, I'll do better next time," this perseverance to try and try again will contribute to your happiness.

Another so-called secret of life is that laughter is the best medicine to live's aches and pains. And, the best kind of laughter is laughing at yourself, because in addition to becoming happy, you become free.

In closing, don't work to be happy, keep busy so you won't be sad. Enjoy today's happiness. Learn to accept yourself and your faults; this is one of the ways you will discover how to find happiness.

How We Find Happiness in Life

Happiness is life's most desired goal. But we can never achieve it while we continue to look outside of ourselves, as it is an inside job.

"Happiness cannot be traveled to, owned, earned, worn or consumed. Happiness is the spiritual experience of living every minute with love, grace, and gratitude".

Throughout our evolutionary journey, we have tried every strategy imaginable and searched almost everywhere in our quest for true happiness. We have had some great experiences and learned a lot along the way, but we have never found what we are searching for. Eventually, we grow tired of searching and turn our attention to the one place we haven't looked so far; inside ourselves. True happiness is not something that can be sought and acquired; it is our soul's natural state of being, and we can only connect with by going within.

Anything we do, it is simply our inner quality that we are going to spread. We cannot do anything of tremendous value for our planet until anything of accurate value occurs within us. Thus, if we want to be connected to the world, the first thing we must do is to transform ourselves right into a happy being.

It doesn't matter what we do in our lives; whether it is business, studying or giving assistance to someone or some cause, we're doing it because deep down, it gives us satisfaction. Each activity that every individual executes on this globe rises from a desire. We were not unhappy when we were a child, as joy and happiness is a source which resides within each one of us. So all we have to do is to go for it and take charge of that joy which is residing in us.

Everything in the universe is in order. The sun comes wonderfully well up in the sky. The flowers flourish beautifully, no stars fall along, and the galaxies are functioning perfectly. Today, the whole cosmos is occurring divinely well, but just a negative thought is warming up on our brain enables us to believe that today is a poor day.

Suffering occurs basically when most human beings shed perception in regards to what this life is all about. Our emotional process becomes far larger than the existential procedure, or our petty creation becomes far more critical compared to GOD's Creations, to place it bluntly. This is the way to obtain all suffering. We miss the complete sense of what this means to be alive here. An emotion within us or thought within our mind establishes the nature of the experience right now. And our thought may have nothing to accomplish even with the restricted reality of our lifestyle. The entire creation is happening beautifully well, but just one considered emotion can ruin everything.

Anything we consider as "our mind" isn't ours. It is merely society's empty talk. Everyone and anyone whom we encounter on a daily base put some idea or information in our head, and we truly have no choice about whose idea we accept or don't accept. This information is advantageous once we learn HOW TO process them and use them. This accumulation of opinions and information that we collect is simply useful for our survival on the planet. It is not something related to who we are.

Life is about learning and appreciating what GOD has created for us on this plant. It is not about twisting and distorting it. When we rely on the external situation to make us joyful and content, we could never feel true happiness. The quality of our life doesn't depend on what car we drive, how much money we have in a bank account, or how big our house is, but how content and happy we feel inside.

Although each one of us is unique, and what works for one may not for others, but there are simply areas that tend to make a big difference to people's happiness in life, and crucially they are all areas that are within our control:

1 - Care for others genuinely: Caring genuinely for others around us is essential to our happiness. Being caring means wishing the best for others, and acknowledging in them the same wants, needs, aspirations, and even fears that we have too. It means providing a listening ear, noticing when someone needs help, and helping our community without asking for a reward. Being caring allows us to have empathy for others and to live a life based on affection, love, and compassion for the people around us.

2 - Connect with people: "Happiness is influenced not only by the people you know but by the people they know." This means that by surrounding ourselves with happier people we become happier, we make the people close to us happier and make the people close to them happier. People with strong and vast social relationships are happier, healthier and live longer. A close relationship with family and friends brings love, compassion, meaning and belonging into our lives and grow our sense of self-worth. "To touch the soul of another human being is to walk on holy ground" ~ Stephen Covey

3 - Notice the world around you: Taking Notice is about observing those things that we find beautiful and being mindful of them in our daily life. It can be easy to rush through life without stopping to notice much. Paying more attention to the present moment, to our thoughts and feelings, and the world around us; can improve our wellbeing. Becoming more aware of the present moment not only help us to enjoy the world around us more and understand ourselves better, but also recognize anew things that we have been taking for granted.

4 - Have something to look forward to Happiness in anticipation is the key here. By having something to look forward to, no matter how our situations, bring happiness into our lives, well before the circumstance happened. If your life is a series of undesirable duties, commitments, and unpleasant tasks, take some time to find out something that YOU would find enjoyable. And make time to do it. "Happiness is the anticipation and the realization of the fulfillment of a dream."

5 - Avoid false beliefs and expectations: "Our authentic happiness is blocked by our false belief that life should be how we want it to be. The expectation that accompanies this false belief sets us up for disappointment, frustration, anger, and unhappiness". Our expectations create our reality, and they change our lives emotionally and physically. Unreasonable expectations can make life extremely hard and unhappy. These expectations are designed by our ego, as nothing give our ego a stronger sense of self-identity as an experience that supports our sad life-story. "In other words, we unconsciously create expectations so we can feel sad and disappointed when they are not met. Our ego is addicted to sadness and painful emotions". Master to drop all expectations and open your heart, begin to love yourself, and move beyond your ego. Embrace freedom from your ego.

6 - Be comfortable with who you are: Finding ourselves, our authenticity will help us to feel our beauty. When we endeavor to be who we are, to be true to ourselves, and accept ourselves with all our flaws and imperfections, we will automatically feel attractive and unique. Beauty is never dependent upon the approval of others. Quite the contrary, beauty is very much self-defined and self-created. "To be beautiful means to be yourself. You don't need to be accepted by others. You need to accept yourself." ~Thich Nhat Hanh. By accepting ourselves and becoming kinder to ourselves, we will be able to see our shortcomings as opportunities to learn and grow.

7 - Find a purpose in life: We all have intact potential, perhaps even areas of intelligence, to become something entirely different, or somehow more than what we appear to be right now. People who find meaning and purpose in their lives are happier, feel more in control and get more out of what they do. They become less stressed, anxious, or depressed. But how do we find meaning and purpose in life? We're all wired differently. Some of us feel more connected to nature; others find meaning by employing in nurturing. The key is to know what works for us. Learning to live our purpose is essentially a spiritual exercise and an inside job. Search how and what give you that sense of fulfillment and deep connection, and then peruse it in all that you do.

8 - Train yourself to be more positive: There is a positive aspect in everything, in every person, in every situation. Sometimes it's not obvious, and we have to look hard. Even when we are faced with a difficult situation, we can think to ourselves "What is good about this?" No matter how unpleasant the circumstance might look, we always can find something good if we take the time to think about it. Everything, good or bad is a learning experience. And there is always a lesson to be gained from every bad experience. "There are moments when troubles enter our lives, and we can do nothing to avoid them. But they are there for a reason. Only when we have overcome them will we understand why they were there" ~ Paulo Coelho

9 - Live Mindfully: "Life is not what it's supposed to be. It's what it is. The way you cope with it is what makes the difference" ~ Virginia Satir. Life is full of challenges. The way we manage them can make a difference between whether we let them control our lives, or we find a way to embrace every challenge as it arises. By practicing mindfulness, we can find a more empowering way to react to the challenges life brings us. It also helps us to train our mind, manage our thoughts and feelings, and reduce stress and anxiety.

10 - Take care of your body: "Your body is precious. It is our vehicle for awakening. Treat it with care." ~Buddha. There is a powerful mind-body connection through which emotional, mental, social, spiritual, and behavioral factors can directly affect our health. Being active makes us happier as well as healthier. By spending time outdoors, eating healthy foods, and getting enough sleep, we can improve our wellbeing. A serene mind is nothing without a healthy body to carry it, so show your body the same compassion that you show everyone, by taking care of it.

It is positive time now that we look inside ourselves and see HOW TO produce personal wellbeing. From our own experience of life, we can observe that wellbeing will come to us when we change our perception of life. We need to realize if we are determined to create our happiness and wellbeing by the outside factors it will never happen. As nothing will be %100 the way, we want them to be. When we accept this fact, then we will be able to work on ourselves as an individual to become the person we want to be. And happiness will be our only choice which has been our authentic nature by creation in the first place. "Focus on the journey, not the destination. Joy is found not in finishing an activity but in doing it." ~ Greg Anderson

Printed in Poland
by Amazon Fulfillment
Poland Sp. z o.o., Wrocław